THE DOCTOR IS IN

The
DOCTOR
IS IN

A 7-Step Prescription
for Optimal Wellness

TRAVIS L. STORK, MD

with William Doyle

GALLERY
BOOKS

A Division of Simon & Schuster
New York   London   Toronto   Sydney

Gallery Books
A Division of Simon & Schuster, Inc.
1230 Avenue of the Americas
New York, NY 10020

First Gallery Books trade paperback edition April 2011

GALLERY BOOKS and colophon are trademarks of Simon & Schuster, Inc.

For information about special discounts for bulk purchases, please contact Simon & Schuster Special Sales at 1-866-506-1949 or business@simonandschuster.com.

The Simon & Schuster Speakers Bureau can bring authors to your live event. For more information or to book an event contact the Simon & Schuster Speakers Bureau at 1-866-248-3049 or visit our website at www.simonspeakers.com.

Designed by Level C, Inc.

Manufactured in the United States of America

10   9   8   7   6   5   4   3   2   1

The Library of Congress cataloged the hardcover as follows:

Stork, Travis.
   The doctor is in : a 7-step prescription for optimal wellness / by Travis L. Stork with William Doyle.
      p.   cm.
   1. Health.   2. Medicine, Popular.   I. Doyle, William, 1957–   II. Title.
RA776.S883 2010
   613—dc22   2010005746

ISBN 978-1-4391-6740-3
ISBN 978-1-4391-6742-7 (pbk)
ISBN 978-1-4391-6743-4 (ebook)

To my family and friends,
who make me the luckiest man alive

Contents

Note to the Reader

This publication is intended to provide helpful and informative material on the subjects addressed. It is sold with the understanding that the authors and publisher are not engaged in rendering medical, mental health, or any other kind of personal professional services in the book.

The reader should consult his or her medical, mental health, or other competent professional before adopting any of the suggestions in this book or drawing inferences from it.

This book is not intended in any way to be a substitute for professional medical or health advice, diagnosis, or treatment. Never disregard professional medical or health advice or delay seeking it because of something you have read in this or any other book.

The authors and publisher specifically disclaim all responsibility for any liability, injury, loss or risk, personal or otherwise, which is incurred as a consequence, directly or indirectly, of the use and application of any of the contents of this book.

Introduction

I believe in keeping things simple.

If there's one way to describe how I try to live my life, it's this: simply healthy. Good health does not need to be overly complex. I don't believe in crazy, extreme diets or health fads. I'm not big on long lists of health rules. I don't believe you need to be an elite athlete to enjoy the many benefits of a healthy body. I'm healthy and I certainly don't diet—and I am far from an elite athlete!

I'm also very skeptical of any health authority who behaves like he or she has all the answers.

But one thing I do know is that the information in these pages, when you put it into action, will improve your life and help you conquer disease before it happens, and it can radically change your physical life for the better.

This book will put you on an easy to follow path to optimal wellness, a path you'll never want to leave. It will help you realize that every day, you embark on a personal voyage involving your health and wellness. After all, it is the series of choices, attitudes, and decisions we make each and every day that directly affect how good we feel and how well we live—today, tomorrow, and for the rest of our lives. You'll also learn how to deal with being bombarded daily with a bewildering array of medical theories, health information, and "expert" opinions, which too often make the journey not only seem overwhelmingly difficult and complex, but incredibly stressful and confusing. I'll crack the total code of wellness for you from the per-spective of a medical doctor who has treated thousands of patients and who knows what it takes to enjoy optimal wellness. And I prom-ise you that I won't ask you to do anything that I wouldn't do in my own life.

I realize that this may seem like a lot to deliver. But again, I believe that achieving good health is truly simple. In fact, I've broken down the main components to becoming healthy into seven very simple, powerful, and positive steps:

TRAVIS L. STORK, MD

R̵   **DR. STORK'S 7-STEP PRESCRIPTION FOR OPTIMAL WELLNESS**

1. Be Your Own Health Guru.
2. Eat to Savor Life.
3. Give Your Body a Daily Vacation.
4. Nail Your Health Stats.
5. Master the Medical Process.
6. Open Your Mind to Alternatives.
7. Make the Mind-Body Connection.

As you can tell from the prescription, this is not a book of "alternative medicine." It is not a book based on a hunch, a theory, a proprietary concept or secret formula of mine, or a few small clinical trials on nervous lab rats. There are no rigid rules to follow and no impossible targets to hit.

This book is based not only on my years of medical training and practice, but on the latest, hard-core, evidence-based breakthrough research, the kind that is peer-reviewed and published in respected scientific and medical journals. Using my professional experience and personal experiences as a patient, I will tackle the most life-changing medical topics and breakthroughs for you, and illuminate the basic foundations of your good health. I will break it all down for you, demystifying and debunking as I go, and I'll show you how to navigate your way to making the healthiest choices and taking the positive steps that will fill you with strength, energy, and total wellness.

The very first step is realizing that you have the power to completely transform your health through a few simple, crucial actions that can change your life. Now let's put that power into action!

ONE

BE YOUR OWN HEALTH GURU

"Doctor, don't let my son die," a frantic man with a little boy in his arms said to me as he ran into the ER. He laid the boy down on a gurney. "Please save him!"

I noted that his son was blue and barely breathing.

It was midnight on my first shift as a full-fledged emergency room doctor. I was a young physician in training at Vanderbilt University Medical Center in Nashville, and I was working my first-ever shift completely on my own, moonlighting in a small ER in a remote little town in Tennessee. I had confidence in my skills and training, but it was an incredibly scary experience to know that for the first time ever, I was solo and had no backup. Until this particular night I had always been under the supervision of an attending physician, but now I was completely on my own.

Until that moment it had been a quiet night, punctuated only by the sounds of the cleaning crew, the vending machines, and the beeps of hospital equipment. I was partway through a twenty-four-hour shift, and feeling good since nothing catastrophic had happened.

As I looked at the boy, who was helpless and at the edge of death, I felt an overwhelming sense of responsibility and dread, accompanied by an adrenaline rush from having the opportunity to put my skills to the test. It was a feeling no amount of medical training could have prepared me for. I thought, *This is where the rubber meets the road.*

My brain switched into my doctor's autopilot mode, a hyper-focused state of mind that happens when I'm faced with a very sick patient in a crisis and the clock is ticking. As a nurse pulled a crash cart of emergency tools and equipment over to the boy, I repeated a simple mantra to myself, "A, B, C"—the basic CPR drill of check the airway (A), check breathing (B), and check circulation (C). They're the first steps I take with every sick patient I see, and it's a sequence of action that's been burned into my brain since Day 1 of medical school.

The child was unconscious and making some labored attempts at breathing, but he was not protecting his airway—he did not have a gag reflex, which is an involuntary safety response our throat uses to prevent aspiration.

I realized we had to address the unprotected airway first. I quickly checked his pulse. It was faint and very fast. In my mind I chanted another refrain: "IV-O2-monitor . . . IV-O2-monitor." Still on autopilot, I knew what I had to do: start an intravenous line, place an oxygen mask on the boy, and hook him up to an ECG monitor.

But before I could, the boy stopped breathing completely.

I squeezed a bag-valve mask over his nose and mouth to send oxygen into his lungs so it could then be pumped by his heart to other vital organs, like the brain. In a scenario like this, time is of the essence because a brain without oxygen is facing catastrophic consequences. "Time is brain," the saying goes, meaning that every minute without oxygen means more brain cells die, never to be recovered.

I gathered my airway equipment, checking that everything would work properly. I then checked his blood glucose, which was normal. As I passed the endotracheal tube through his mouth and into his trachea, I could have heard a pin drop. The room was almost deadly quiet, which is exactly what you want as an ER doctor, since unnecessary commotion causes a lot of undue panic. I watched the tube pass down through the young boy's vocal cords and I started squeezing oxygen into his lungs through the artificial breathing tube I'd just placed.

As I worked, the boy's father was standing in the corner of the room in a state of complete disbelief. I kept talking to him, trying to figure out what might have happened, all the while attempting to reassure him that we would do everything we could for his son.

"Do you have any medicines in the house?" I asked the father as I simultaneously analyzed the ECG, or electrocardiogram, that traced the heart's electrical rhythm. "Could he have swallowed some?" We were able to figure out that the boy had gotten into his family's medicine chest and had likely taken what should have been a fatal overdose of antidepressants. That discovery was absolutely crucial to figuring out how to treat him.

Fortunately, I was able to stabilize the child's condition. Soon thereafter, we airlifted him by helicopter to a larger medical center. Four days later the little boy left the hospital without any residual effects from his overdose.

Looking back on it, I see this event as the moment in my life when I truly began to see myself as a doctor; up until that point people called me Dr. Stork, but I didn't really feel like an MD. Such events are incredibly exhilarating but also quite scary. That's life in the emergency department. Along with the absolutely mind-blowing feeling of saving someone's life, moments later you may have to tell a wife that her husband has just died. I'll never do anything in my life that comes close to rivaling the challenges of being a good doctor, which is why I have so much respect for my peers in the world of medicine. It truly is a one-of-a-kind job.

As an emergency medicine doctor, I'm able to help people who are confronted with acute and sudden medical challenges, often with a "ticking clock" counting down quickly toward very severe consequences, including permanent injury and death. In a sense, all of medicine is potentially emergency medicine. But as an emergency room specialist, I get to develop expertise across an incredibly wide spectrum of medical subjects, which is one of the features I love about it as a profession.

It definitely isn't always pleasant in the ER. I've had patients physically attack me, projectile-vomit on me more times than I'd like to remember, and I once had an intoxicated gang leader assault me with the very suture needle that I was using to repair a wound he had sustained in the previous night's gang battle. In the typical emergency department, patients are often lined up in hallways, and it can be pure chaos. Sometimes people come into the ER too late to be saved and they die in my arms. But the good far outweighs the bad, and the variety of experiences in the ER is like nothing else.

Being an ER doctor is my dream job, but I'm lucky to have two more responsibilities that I absolutely love. As a member of Vanderbilt University's faculty, I get to teach medical students and resident physicians in training. I was blessed to have many incredible teachers along the way, and now I'm able to pass on the lessons I've learned to future generations of doctors and see them begin their life's mission to improve medical care for everyone. I love seeing the passion of the medical students and residents working at Vanderbilt. These are some of the nation's brightest minds and they chose medicine because they want to help people.

And as host of the daily TV series *The Doctors,* a program devoted to bringing the best medical and health information to our viewers, I, along with a panel of other doctors, get to go on TV every day to talk about health and wellness. The success we've achieved so far— strong ratings, critical acclaim—is a perfect illustration of how much we all want the best, most cutting-edge information to help us live the healthiest lives we can. People have a real thirst for accessible and reliable health information.

I didn't plan on a TV career. First and foremost I'm a doctor, and I plan on staying that way. I'd never been in front of a camera until my final year of residency. Through a series of accidental coincidences a number of years ago, I wound up appearing on the TV show, *The Bachelor: Paris,* which at the time I figured was a unique, you-only-live-once type of experience. Then I got a call from the *Dr. Phil* show to contribute regular medical segments to the program, which I really enjoyed. Later, when Jay McGraw developed the concept for *The Doctors,* he asked me to host the show along with obstetrician and gynecologist Dr. Lisa Masterson, plastic surgeon and reconstructive surgery expert Dr. Andrew Ordon, and pediatrician Dr. James Sears.

You know what clinched the deal for me? When Dr. Phil told me that I could educate more people, in terms of sheer numbers, in a one-hour episode of *The Doctors,* than in my entire career in the ER. Also, my boss, the chairman of the Emergency Medicine Department at Vanderbilt, Dr. Corey Slovis, has always encouraged me to "show people what emergency medicine is really all about."

In a sense, it all started for me that day in the ER with the boy who took the overdose of antidepressants. The way his father looked at me, I knew he trusted me with his son's life, and that made me realize how much responsibility I have as a doctor. In that moment I was the most important medical authority and the greatest health guru on Earth to that man and his little boy.

But here's an amazing idea, something you may not realize yet and should cause you, to some extent, to feel the same way I did in the ER that day: you have as much power over your health as I had with that child. I am convinced that secret can change your life. In fact, the power I held at that moment in time over that boy's life is only a fraction of the power you hold in your grasp every single day of your life to affect your own medical destiny, your ability to achieve optimal health. It's true. *The power you have over your own health is potentially thousands of times stronger than that of any doctor. The most powerful health guru in history is you.*

How strong is this power? In health there are no guarantees, but consider this: by making a few simple "tweaks" to your lifestyle and the way you think, steps I will outline in the pages that follow, you can work to achieve these potential flesh-and-blood medical miracles for yourself:

- You have the power to make changes that may extend your life span by up to a decade or more.

- You have the power to potentially avoid the great majority of chronic diseases.

- You have the power to slash your risk of developing cardiovascular disease.

- You have the power to lower your high blood pressure.

- You have the power to slow or prevent the onset of type 2 diabetes.

- You have the power to reduce your risk of certain cancers.

- You have the power to conquer and reverse obesity.

- You have the power to reduce your risk of osteoarthritis, erectile dysfunction, osteoporosis, and macular degeneration.

- You have the power to avoid many years and countless thousands of dollars' worth of agonizing medical crises and procedures, hospital stays, and medications due to preventable conditions.

- You have the power to transform your health and the health of your family.

- You may even have the power in some cases to delay the onset or reduce your risk of Alzheimer's disease.

Have you ever heard of any doctor and/or pill on earth with a fraction of this power? This spectacular power is already in your hands, just waiting to be unleashed. That's what this book is about—how to identify your power over your health, sharpen it, and unleash it.

ASK DR. STORK

Question: My family has a history of diabetes and heart disease. How can I improve my health, and why should I even bother, when I'm genetically predisposed to these illnesses? Isn't health largely genetic?

Answer: Family history can definitely be a risk factor for chronic disease, and there are illnesses that are both inherited and manifested primarily through genetics. But genes have been estimated to account for only 30 percent of preventable deaths. In many instances, genetics only "loads the gun" of potential disease, and your behavior and/or environment "pulls the trigger" for it to be activated. In most cases, chronic diseases are initiated and fueled over time by the interplay between genetic, environmental, and behavioral factors, such as your diet and physical activity.

The biggest proportional contributor to premature death in the United States is our personal behavior—including what we eat and don't eat, how much physical activity we get, and whether or not we smoke.

The good news is that strong evidence, from many sources, links most chronic disease to the wrong dietary patterns and physical inactivity. So if you improve those factors, you can often prevent disease from manifesting.

Actually, that is spectacular news!

WHY YOU MUST BE YOUR OWN HEALTH GURU

The health care system is broken—and won't be fixed any time soon. Therefore, we must take charge of our own health, right now, this very second.

We are largely the masters of our own health universe. But as a society, we seem to be doing some things awfully wrong, and we are paying an increasingly terrible price, both as a nation and as individuals.

A huge factor is that we don't teach health in our medical schools. Instead, we teach a patchwork of disease management. Care to know how much time was spent in my medical training on healthy lifestyles and prevention? Essentially none.

"Our society is at war," declared one panel of experts in the February 2000 edition of the *Journal of Applied Physiology*. "Although it may not be commonly publicized in this manner, make no mistake, our society, and even the world's population in general, is truly at war against a common enemy. That enemy is modern chronic disease."

Chronic diseases are the most common cause of preventable death in the nation. These are diseases that progress slowly and continue for a long time, including cardiovascular disease (such as coronary artery disease, heart failure, hypertension, and stroke), obesity, type 2 diabetes, some cancers, and osteoporosis.

Diet, Exercise, and Health

A few years ago, two experts at UCLA, Christian K. Roberts and R. James Barnard, were invited by the *Journal of Applied Physiology* to review the entire universe of medical and scientific evidence on the connections between diet, exercise, and health. Their conclusions, published in 2005 in an article titled "Effects of Exercise and Diet on Chronic Disease," which I'll summarize here, are startling, and of tremendous importance to your health:

The evidence is overwhelming that your diet and the amount of physical activity you engage in can reduce the risk of developing numerous chronic diseases, including coronary artery disease, hypertension, diabetes, and metabolic syndrome, and can even reverse existing disease.

Also, the risk of several other chronic diseases may be reduced by physical activity and diet, including several forms of cancer, osteoporosis, arthritis, stroke and congestive heart failure, chronic renal [kidney] failure, Alzheimer's disease, and erectile dysfunction.

Consider the implications of these findings—your personal attitude and personal choices can optimize your health by helping you conquer a host of illnesses before they happen, including the biggest killers in America: heart disease, cancer, and diabetes.

Now, that's power!

Americans spend over $2 trillion a year on health care. Ninety-five percent of that goes to medical care of sickness that's already struck us—and only 5 percent is spent on prevention! As Senator Tom Harkin quipped, "We currently do not have a health care system in the United States; we have a sick care system." He's absolutely right.

While I am astonished at the amazing technology and capabilities of American medicine, you and I can't rely on the health care system alone to control our destinies. We have fantastic doctors and nurses in this country, but the overall system is broken. Here are some of the nightmare consequences of our thoroughly convoluted and mismanaged non-system:

- The U.S. spends the most money on health care of any country on earth—yet ranks toward the bottom of developed nations on quality of care, and thirty-seventh among all nations, on par with Serbia.

- Among developed nations, the U.S. ranks near the bottom on most standard measures of health status. We spend two times more money per person as European nations, yet we are twice as sick from chronic diseases.

- Childhood obesity is becoming a national epidemic and is threatening the health of millions of kids. The number of obese American children and adolescents has tripled in the last twenty years. By the year 2015, two in every five adults and one in every four children in the United States may be obese. Only one-third of Americans are in the "healthy weight" category.

- More than half of Americans over fifty have diabetes, high blood pressure, heart disease, or some other chronic condition. In fact, obesity, diabetes, and hypertension are becoming commonplace even in children.

- About 250,000 deaths per year are caused primarily by a lack of physical activity.

- 150,000 new cases of colon cancer are diagnosed every year and 56,000 people die from it. But only 52 percent of patients are screened for the disease.

- Asthma causes about 500,000 hospitalizations every year, yet only about 28 percent of patients get a comprehensive management plan from their clinician.

This isn't your fault, or your doctor's fault. It's the system's fault, and society's fault. And it doesn't look like the health care system will be truly fixed anytime soon. But for you and your family, there is a solution to this mess, and a clue to it lies in the place where I work.

THE SECRET OF THE ER:
A TALE OF THREE PATIENTS

I'll never go out of business as an ER doctor. As long as things go wrong in life, and until everyone takes perfect care of themselves, there will always be a need for emergency medicine.

Do you know what the most common problem I see is? I'll give you a hint: it's not gunshot wounds, car accidents, household accidents, or domestic violence—though I regularly treat all of these.

The biggest problem driving many of my patients into the emergency room these days is the damage they are doing their own bodies, over time, by making the wrong choices.

It may be hard to believe, but poor choices over time are what's injuring and killing hundreds of thousands of Americans every year. What I see most in the ER is the acute worsening of a multitude of chronic conditions like heart disease, diabetes, and obesity, which are largely self-inflicted and driven by voluntary lifestyle choices. It is a slow, painful, American mass-suicide driven by bad food choices and lack of physical activity. It's a special problem in places like Tennessee, where I work, where sedentary lifestyles and overeating are at crisis levels and the rate of obesity is skyrocketing even faster than the national average. You can't really blame many of these people. The unfortunate fact is that as a nation we haven't fully woken up to the links between lifestyle and chronic disease. The things I see in the ER are a constant reminder of how poorly we take care of ourselves in this country.

I confess, I consider myself a happy, well-adjusted guy, but the ER can sometimes be a sad and frustrating place to work. It's not just because people frequently die there, but how chronic disease can force people to live—at the mercy of medicines, doctor visits, and ongoing physical and mental pain. No matter how positive their outlook is on life, once they're in a body that no longer functions well, it can be such a grind.

Many Americans who are only in their fifties or sixties—and even younger—are being forced to take an endless grand tour of doctor's offices and pharmacies when they should be enjoying themselves and their families instead.

Let me tell you about three types of patients I've seen in the last year. These are not real names. They are composite characters, and absolutely typical of the patients I see all the time in the ER:

=========

First there's Ruth. She's only fifty-six years old, but she looks like she could be in her eighties. She's already had two heart attacks. She is sixty pounds overweight. Like many Americans she drifted into the obese category of weight over the years by eating too much of the wrong foods and rarely getting any meaningful physical activity. Ruth's primary source of nourishment for the past twenty-five years or more has been supersized fast food, chips and unhealthy snacks, ice cream, and soda. A victim of the unhealthy aspects of American food culture, she never learned about healthy eating and exercise in a way that she could put into action.

At an age when Ruth should be thriving, she has already developed heart disease, obesity, type 2 diabetes, osteoarthritis, high blood pressure, a peptic ulcer, fibromyalgia, and recurring urinary tract infections, one of which led to a long stay in the ICU due to something called septic shock after the infection invaded her bloodstream. Did I mention her feet are numb as a symptom of her diabetes? She once stepped on a nail and because she couldn't feel it, she developed a severe infection leading to partial amputation of her foot. On top of all of that, she is clinically depressed, which is completely understandable, given her other conditions.

Ruth is on over a dozen different medications. (This is not unusual at all—these days I'm seeing patients with medication lists that are twenty-plus deep. I know it sounds crazy, but it's true.) Her body is starting a full-scale collapse, and a cascade of self-inflicted health problems is overwhelming her.

Last week was an average one for Ruth. It was filled up with scheduled doctor visits. She saw her primary care doctor on Monday, the cardiologist on Tuesday, and the kidney specialist for tests on Wednesday. She contracted the flu over the weekend, got dehydrated, and was rushed to the ER with acute renal failure. We wound up having to put her on dialysis.

When I saw Ruth on her last ER visit, I got incredibly frustrated, even angry—though I never let on. Not at her, but because somehow, as a society, we've failed to help her stop this series of disasters before they happened. Instead of savoring a happy, physically active life, she is becoming a prisoner of her illnesses, most of which were avoidable. Whenever I think about cutting corners in my own life and feel myself being lured into the trap of becoming a couch potato on a steady diet of fast food or overly processed chain restaurant meals, I think of Ruth. A lifetime of all-you-can-eat buffets isn't so appealing when you consider the consequences.

———

The next patient is Frank, a sixty-year-old man who represents how Ruth's life may end up in just a few years.

Frank was captain of the high school football team, a star quarterback, and a superstar in his early adult life. He became a successful insurance executive, and eventually his routine became very sedentary, based on desk work and driving his car. He didn't find time to exercise, because he was always "too busy."

After dinner most nights, he plopped down on his fully equipped reclining chair and watched an average of three or four hours of TV. He developed a long love affair with cigarettes and fast-food cheeseburgers. Like Ruth, he became obese and in his case, put on a gigantic potbelly from years of large portions of unhealthy eating. And also like Ruth, he developed lifestyle-driven chronic diseases that cascaded upon each other.

But unlike Ruth, who can still get around on her own, Frank is now largely bedridden, and instead of living with his family, he is in an assisted-living facility, which operates much like a nursing home. He needs assistance just keeping track of when to take the right pill from his enormous supply of medications. When he does get out of bed, Frank is confined to a wheelchair. I can't tell you how often I see people who, like Frank, are in wheelchairs, not because they have a physical injury, but because they've been physically inactive and/or obese for so long that their bodies become unable to support them in the simple act of walking.

Recently, Frank was experiencing severe chest pain and was brought to the hospital. It turns out he was suffering from a massive heart attack. Frank's wife approached me after we urgently sent him for a cardiac catheterization and said, "I tried to get him to quit smoking for years, and he just wouldn't listen." We were able to save him that day, but who knows what is in store for him in the months and years ahead.

At this point, there is no way to "fix" Frank because the damage is already done. As Dr. Michael Weitzman of NYU's Langone Medical Center once said, "It's a lot easier not to develop problems than it is to cure them." The medical system will do everything in its power to keep Frank alive as long as possible, but his capacity for independent living and a long, vibrant life is essentially gone.

I once heard a doctor say, "You're only as young as your oldest body part," which I'm afraid is quite true. If, like Frank, at the age of sixty you suffer a heart attack and your heart is basically that of an eighty-five-year-old, I hate to break it to you, but your life expectancy is probably going to be dictated by your oldest body part. That's why it is so essential to take great care of yourself before it's too late. What happened to Ruth and Frank is happening to countless people all across America, all the time.

I tell you this not so you give up hope, but to inspire you. Because there is a silver lining to all this: it absolutely, positively doesn't have to be your fate. You have the power to completely transform your own health—by taking a few simple steps.

––––––

Take the case of the third patient I'll tell you about, whom I'll call George, a man I saw in the ER for an easily treated sprained ankle. He is ninety-three years old and in excellent shape. He lives independently, chops wood, takes regular power walks, and goes fishing with his buddies when he's not chasing his great-grandkids around.

Almost forty years ago, when he was in his fifties, George got a huge wake-up call. He was diagnosed with diabetes, and his doctor told him that if he didn't make major improvements to his lifestyle, he might not live that long or may end up with a low quality of life. George was stunned by the diagnosis, and he decided to immediately take charge. Over the next four decades he woke up every morning and resolved to optimize his health. He worked out, took his medications, and ate healthy meals while allowing himself regular treats and indulgences. He made health his hobby, and he had fun while doing it.

In short, he became his own health guru.

––––––

Only you, working in partnership with your doctor, can sift through the universe of good and bad health information, tailor it to your own medical history and health conditions, and take positive action to optimize your health.

What does it mean to be optimizing your health? It means:

- Staying out of hospitals and emergency rooms, by preventing the need for you to ever go there.

- Taking as few medications as possible, or none at all.

- Thriving physically and living your healthiest possible life.

- Feeling strong and powerful every day of your life.

You can achieve all of this—if you decide right now to become your own health guru. You have the power to save your life and shape your physical destiny every day by the decisions you make.

HOW TO BE YOUR OWN HEALTH GURU

In America, we love health gurus.

There seems to be an endless supply of them in the media, and you see them everywhere from *The Oprah Winfrey Show, Larry King Live*, and the *Today* show to PBS fundraisers and late-night informercials.

Some health gurus are household names. Some are medical doctors, though many are not, and some are celebrities with no real medical knowledge or training whatsoever. Some have excellent advice on healthy living, but others are outright quacks, dispensing advice that is not based on scientific evidence.

Celebrities can be passionate and articulate health gurus, and it's especially easy for them to step into the national spotlight to argue their theories. But there's nothing about celebrities that gives them any authority whatsoever to speak about health and medicine, other than what they've learned through their own reading and research, which may or may not have any value for you. It's a big problem in our society, that people can be more inclined to listen to celebrity figures than they are to people who give better information based on real evidence. Celebrities shouldn't be your health gurus—you should be your own. By all means, listen to their ideas if you like. But before you adopt anyone's advice, put their ideas to the test by doing your own research and talking to your own doctor.

Another common source of misinformation are the health experts in one field who offer advice in an area they're completely unqualified to comment on. For instance, your yoga instructor should not be your main source of advice when it comes to your medications. The health gurus you meet in daily life—your brother-in-law, a fellow mom in the playground, the salesclerk in the health food store—can also be problematic. They, too, can have both great health ideas and bad ones.

How to Get Your Friends and Family to Support You

When you decide to make health your hobby and you commit to optimize your health, it helps tremendously to have friends and family who support you. This isn't always easy. Your spouse may be dedicated to an unhealthy lifestyle and show no signs of wanting to change. Or your friends may try to undermine you in subtle ways and make fun of your health hobby. (They may be doing it out of jealousy, secretly wishing that they had the same amount of dedication.) Remember, it's hard to convince people to change, and it's not your job necessarily to change your spouse.

If you have a friend or significant other who's not going to support you as you strive to optimize your health, I don't think you should shut them out of your life. But you need to tell them point-blank not to bring you down in your pursuit of this new goal of living a healthy life. Make it clear that you don't appreciate them making fun of you or being critical of your new food and exercise choices. Better yet, have them browse this book and they'll realize there are no rigid rules and no impossible targets to prevent them from optimizing their own health.

Another group to be wary of: "health nuts." You may know the kind of person I'm talking about—they eat only nuts, twigs, sprouts, berries, and organic vegetable juice. This is a tough model to follow because there's a fine line between health conscious and flat-out health nut. The last thing you should do is go crazy over your health. If you're driving yourself to distraction trying to be healthy, then you're not being healthy. You should take a sane and relaxed approach, and realize that the key steps to optimal health are surprisingly simple. Make health your hobby, not an obsession. You should enjoy a healthy lifestyle, but it doesn't have to be an extreme ascetic lifestyle devoid of fun and indulgences.

I'm skeptical of extreme "health fiends." They're often way too skinny, and they've got long lists of foods that are forbidden and "poison." Ironically, some of their ideas are rooted in good science—like the idea that veggies, fruit, and whole grains are crucial to good health. But they've taken these ideas to ridiculous extremes, through wacky theories and rules on eating and cooking that are not based on any real research.

I take health very seriously but I'm not a fanatic about it. I think a big part of health is learning to indulge yourself in the right doses. In fact, occasionally enjoying something that you know isn't perfectly healthy for you is being healthy. It's called sanity!

The bottom line is you alone are the CEO of your own health. The secret is figuring out what to believe, and that is what I plan to teach you. And always remember that what is good for someone else may not be good for you. No one person, and no one guru, should know as much about your health as you. You should have a healthy skepticism about all health information that is given in absolutes, even that offered by a doctor. I know I don't have all the answers. When it comes to your health, nothing is guaranteed and there are no promises. The human body is complex, and people respond differently to different treatments.

TRAVIS L. STORK, M.D.

℞ ## BE YOUR OWN HEALTH GURU

- Decide that you are the CEO of your own health—you are the master of your medical destiny.
- Realize that you don't need to follow a multitude of health crazes, diets, and fads.
- Understand that the most powerful steps to optimal health are surprisingly simple.
- Be open-minded, but also skeptical and demanding of all health experts and information.
- Embrace the power of knowing that one of the ultimate steps to nurture, empower, pamper, and liberate yourself every day is to optimize your health.
- Make health your hobby, not an obsession.
- Work with your doctor to determine the best plan for improving your health.

Once you commit to these steps, you can add years or even decades to your life, conquer sickness before it happens, and feel fantastic. The key is for you to make a serious mental commitment to live a healthy life, and realize that you often can't control life circumstances, but you can always control how you treat your body. It all starts with that mental commitment.

THE TOP 5 WEB SHORTCUTS TO HELP
YOU OPTIMIZE YOUR HEALTH

*Including Dr. Stork's #1 "BI
(Bad Information) Detector"*

1. MedlinePlus: http://medlineplus.gov

MedlinePlus is a gold mine of expert information from the world's largest medical library, the National Library of Medicine (NLM); the National Institutes of Health (NIH); and other government agencies and health-related organizations. The site has extensive information on over 750 diseases and conditions, information on drugs and clinical trials, an illustrated medical encyclopedia, interactive patient tutorials, and a daily ticker of the latest health news. There is no advertising, and MedlinePlus does not endorse any company or product. This should be your go-to site to gather the best health and medical information.

Related sites:

Healthfinder: www.healthfinder.gov

Agency for Healthcare Research and Quality: www.ahrq.gov/consumer/

These are gateway sites of resources and tools on a wide range of health topics, culled from over 1,600 government and nonprofit organizations. They are run by the U.S. government and do not accept advertising.

2. American Institute for Cancer Research: www.aicr.org

American Diabetes Association: www.diabetes.org

American Heart Association: www.americanheart.org

These nonprofit organizations have excellent fact sheets and tips on nutrition, lifestyle, and prevention that will help you reduce your risk for developing cancer, diabetes, and heart disease. You'll notice that many of these tips overlap, which is great news—with a handful of tips you put into action, you're reducing your risks for multiple diseases!

3. WebMD: www.webmd.com/

Emedicine by WebMD: http://emedicine.medscape.com/

WebMD and Emedicine are very good sources of news and background briefings on a wide range of health topics. I really like Emedicine as a site for people who want to get information on illnesses they or a family member or friend may have been diagnosed with or that they want more info about. The sites are advertiser supported, but I find them unbiased, user-friendly, and informative.

4. MyPyramid: www.MyPyramid.gov

This is a U.S. government site that features a wealth of information on healthy eating, weight loss, meal planning, and dietary guidelines. I find the current MyPyramid graphic design kind of confusing, but there's still a lot of excellent information throughout this website.

5. PubMed: www.pubmed.gov

This is my #1 filtering tool for cutting through the infinite clutter of health-related research on the internet, much of which is thoroughly bogus, or not supported by evidence other than anecdotes, or is advertising in disguise.

PubMed is a superior resource if you're highly motivated to read real, evidence-based research and the opinions of the most qualified experts. A free index for searching articles in peer-reviewed medical and scientific journals on health, medicine, fitness, and related topics, PubMed often features summaries and abstracts, and in many cases will provide free links to the full original articles. The articles are often pretty technical, but they can provide good discussion points and questions for you and your doctor. It is a government-run site with no ads, and a tutorial is available at http://www.nlm.nih.gov/bsd/disted/pubmedtutorial/

I use this site as my personal BI (Bad Information) Detector. For example, let's say some expert claims the Mediterranean Diet is an excellent dietary pattern. I'll go to PubMed and type in "mediterranean diet" and "review" so I can get "review articles," which are often the biggest, most comprehensive articles on the subject. Then I explore the results and, bingo, find out that it's true—the Mediterranean Diet is one of the very few so-called diets that are backed up by good evidence. Guess what happens when I type in "maple syrup diet," "master cleanse," or "grapefruit diet"? Nothing. Zip. No results. That usually means there's no good research to prove that they work.

So now you know the benefits of becoming your own health guru, and hopefully I've armed you with some great resources and a healthy dose of skepticism.

Now let's tackle the practical aspects of achieving and maintaining good health.

EAT TO SAVOR LIFE

Every time you sit down to eat, you are making a life-changing decision. You are deciding how well you want to live. You are deciding how long you want to live. And you are deciding how good you want to feel, today and for the rest of your life.

In fact, every time you even look at a piece of food, you are gazing at the destiny of your health.

The key to making that vision a desirable one is to decide, right now, to eat to savor life.

I know eating healthy can seem like a tall order, and to prove how vulnerable I am to the allure of junk food, I'll just be honest. Recently, I had brownies and vanilla ice cream for dessert. For dinner, I had cooked myself a healthy spinach-vegetable lasagna with whole grain noodles and low-fat cottage cheese. So for dessert, I figured, "Hey, why not splurge a little—have some brownies!" So I did. I made a batch and they tasted fantastic.

The next morning I was pressed for time and I spotted the jar of leftover brownies in my kitchen.

Usually I make myself a smoothie from frozen berries, whey protein, and yogurt for breakfast. Or if I'm in a real hurry I'll grab a convenient, healthy oatmeal bar on my way out the door. But as I stood admiring the brownies, I thought, "What the heck, a few brownies for breakfast never hurt anyone." So I grabbed two brownies and savored their chocolatey goodness on my way to work. "Now, this is living," I mused.

Here's where the story gets really bad. At lunchtime I stepped into a conference at the medical center. Next to the ham and swiss sandwiches was a tray full of—you guessed it—brownies. I couldn't help myself. A voice inside me said, "Go for it, Travis." And I did.

There I was, a grown man with a medical degree, jonesing for brownies. I'll admit, I've got a brownie problem. When they're put in front of me, I find it hard not to eat them.

Unfortunately, the human body is not well engineered to eat brownies three times in a twelve-hour period, so needless to say, I didn't feel so good that afternoon. To tell you the truth, I felt pretty awful. So I went for a quick workout late in the day and had a very healthy dinner. For the next few weeks, I passed on the brownies, but I'm comfortable with the fact that at some point I will again succumb to a brownie binge.

My point is, we all have our moments of weakness, and doctors can be as vulnerable to bad food and lifestyle habits as everyone else. Maybe even more so given our bizarre schedules and the hectic pace of hospital life.

We can be the worst patients, and we can also be the worst at taking care of ourselves. Just like everyone else, many doctors forget the power they have over their own health.

I know many doctors who are overweight. Even though doctors know firsthand how detrimental being overweight is to a person's health, they can have trouble with obesity. It is not my intention to disparage doctors who happen to be overweight, but instead to highlight how hard it can be to make good lifestyle choices, even for people who should know better.

Here's another example: I recently had a conversation during a shift in the ER with a fellow doctor in his midforties who was also a father. He looked at me and said, "My cholesterol is well over two-fifty and I haven't done anything to correct it." I was upset with him because he has adorable children who would like him to be around for a long time, and I told him so. "You're right," he said sheepishly. "I need to start paying attention to my own health." A few hours later, another doctor said to me, "Hey, Travis, I just picked up a bunch of cheeseburgers and fries before work. Do you want some?" I looked at him and laughed and said, "Do you realize a lot of our patients are here today because they eat fast food like that every day?" He said, "Yeah, but it tastes so good! You've got to have a little fun!" He's right—it does taste good, at first. Then, about twenty minutes later, I always end up feeling sick. Not a good feeling while working in a busy ER!

———

I've never been on a diet. But I am very healthy in the sense that I feel great physically, my health stats are excellent, and my body weight is normal. I believe the two big reasons for this are: (1) I am extremely active and (2) I truly savor eating. Ninety to 95 percent of the time I savor eating by enjoying the most delicious, healthiest foods I can— and for the remaining 5 or 10 percent I allow myself treats, like those brownies or a cheeseburger and fries every now and then.

The fact is that doctors and scientists haven't yet really figured out how to design the perfect weight-loss diet, a diet that would help us reach a perfect weight and optimize our health. No weight-loss diet in the history of mankind has ever been proven to work in a gold-standard, randomized clinical trial that followed people for a reasonably long period of time, say, over five or ten years—because doing such a trial has thus far proven impossible to perform.

The trouble is, scientists haven't yet figured out a way of putting people on different diets and following them over the decades to the clinical endpoint of death. If they did, they could isolate how well the subjects managed to stay on the diets, what the impact of the diets was on their weight and their health, and the progression of different diseases under each diet.

So instead, what the experts try to do is piece together evidence by comparing different patterns of food behavior that occur in different populations, which is called "nutritional epidemiology." They also try to piece evidence together through questionnaires, or food diaries, or clinical studies that are usually conducted with small groups of people for only a year or less. All this research isn't perfect, but it is pointing in some promising new directions. And it turns out there is a pattern of eating that you can start today that can help you lose weight, optimize your health, extend your life, and make you feel great. This plan is not a militaristic regimen of diet rules to make you suffer, but a plan of lifestyle behaviors for you to enjoy.

It's so simple it can be boiled down into three points, three simple steps that encompass almost everything you and your family need to know about healthy eating. The plan is based on the most cutting-edge, breakthrough nutrition research being performed around the world today, by the greatest scientists and doctors on Earth. These are the experts who publish hard-core research in peer-reviewed medical and scientific journals, comparing different populations and multitudes of different foods and ingredients, trying to isolate the most promising lessons for our health. I have synthesized their most important discoveries and conclusions down to a very simple to understand and remember formula.

I call it the Eat to Savor Life Plan.

TRAVIS L. STORK, MD

R̶ THE EAT TO SAVOR LIFE PLAN: THE
ULTIMATE HEALTH OPTIMIZATION DIET

1. Indulge in healthy eating patterns based largely on many
   different kinds of whole veggies and fruit; whole grains; and
   healthy foods like fish, nuts, and beans.
2. Eat less sodium, bad fats, added sugars, and processed
   foods.
3. Shoot for a healthy weight by balancing your calorie budget
   and enjoying at least 30 to 60 minutes of moderate-intensity
   physical activity on most days of the week.

Taken together, these steps can reduce your risk for the great
majority of chronic disease in America today, including cardiovascular disease, obesity, several forms of cancer, type 2 diabetes,
and other conditions, including Alzheimer's disease, erectile dysfunction, osteoporosis, and osteoarthritis.

Three points—it's that simple.

Notice that there are no painful induction phases, detoxing, intestinal cleansing, juice-only fasts, shocking your system, alkaline food
elimination, or other gobbledygook in the plan. No forbidden food
groups or silly food-combining rules either.

The Eat to Savor Life Plan is a sixty-five-word road map that can
save your life, optimize your health, and drastically revolutionize the
way you feel.

Those sixty-five words represent a synthesis of the emerging con-
sensus opinions of the greatest experts in the world about how to
optimize your health. Every family doctor and general practitioner in the United States should hand this plan out—as an actual

prescription—to every one of their patients, every time they see them. If they did, and if patients started implementing these ideas in their own lives, the national health care crisis would shrink to a fraction of its current size, hospitals and ERs would empty out, and instead of being condemned to wheelchairs, doctor's offices, and hospitals by age fifty-five or sixty, millions of Americans would be playing rac-quetball and ballroom dancing well into their nineties.

You should tape up the plan in your kitchen and inside your medi-cine cabinet, and keep a copy in your purse or wallet. Make it a screen saver on your computer. Stick copies of it in your child's lunch box. Remember, these three points can save your life and optimize your health in a revolutionary new direction.

Think of the Eat to Savor Life Plan as a series of eight "big ideas" or "health optimizers" for you to keep in the back of your mind every day. Physical activity is such an important part of it that I practically consider it to be an essential food group. It is so important that I'll devote the entire chapter after this one to it. I'll also cover "balanc-ing your calorie budget" later in this book. But for now I'll stick to revealing the right way to eat.

I guarantee you that I don't actually manage to do all of these every day, but I do keep them in mind as goals that keep me on track overall, on a week to week basis and beyond. That's how you should approach this list, too.

HOW TO EAT TO SAVOR LIFE

Health Optimizer 1: Indulge

I love food and I don't believe in fad diets. I don't have the time to follow all their ridiculous rules, nor do I have the patience to try an endless procession of new diets once my current one failed (which it inevitably would).

I believe the human genome has programmed us to indulge in food, to enjoy it, to pamper and spoil ourselves with it. We were not programmed to starve, deny, and torture ourselves. In fact, those behaviors usually backfire on us—thanks to the way we're hardwired.

The key is to allow ourselves to fall in love with the foods that are really good for us and indulge in them every day. And we shouldn't be afraid to have a chocolate bar or a root beer float or an order of French fries every now and then, as long as we savor the good stuff most of the time and keep track of our portion sizes. The Eat to Savor Life Plan is an "anti-diet": there are no evil or forbidden foods, just some foods to savor more and others to savor less. It requires making food a healthy hobby, not a neurotic obsession.

Most fad diets don't work for long, and in the end, believe it or not, they often make us fat. They cheat us by promising that they'll work, enchanting us with seductive phrases like "Lose 30 pounds in 30 days!" "Fat-burning foods—speed up your metabolism!" "Secret weight-loss supplement—lose 10 pounds without a single crunch!" and "As seen on TV!" Then they rob us when we keep coming back for more, to the tune of $30 billion a year—yes, that's $30 billion that we Americans spend every year in this country on a largely fruitless quest for the perfect diet fad, plan, pill, or shake.

We can lose water weight for a few weeks on a fad diet, or we lose weight briefly because we're being starved of calories. Believe me, it doesn't matter what kinds of foods are being forbidden—when your daily calorie consumption is cut, you'll lose weight. But especially on a fad diet with hard-to-follow rules, the sense of victory we feel after losing ten pounds in two weeks is a false one. As soon as you start eating normally again, you put the weight back on, get frustrated, binge on fattening foods, and wind up worse off than when you started. It's the bounce-back effect. It's real, and it hurts, both physically and psychologically.

There are exceptions to the "diets don't work" rule. Some people can lose weight on a diet or weight loss plan and even keep it off, if the plan offers long-term guidelines and structure to follow. The Weight Watchers program, for example, gets high marks because it is based on healthy eating, controls calories to a reasonable daily amount, and provides a strong support system. And in some cases a diet may help people get a jump start toward a healthier lifestyle. For others, a medically supervised diet may be the only effective solution for addressing problems like morbid obesity and diabetes. But these diets that actually work aren't really diets at all. Rather, they involve a lifestyle change and portion control that bring lasting results.

That is why, as a medical doctor, I hate most diets and diet products. They are designed to steal your money and they aren't based on evidence, just anecdotes. In America, we love to hear dramatic stories like "My brother-in-law lost forty pounds on the Maple Syrup Cleanse!" Well, sure, but where will he be in a month, or a year? Personal stories are fun and, believe me, they sell. But they aren't evidence. They're just, well, stories.

Diets try to bamboozle us with elaborate, scientific-sounding food rules like "Week 1 is the Jump-start Anti-cravings Anti-bloating Phase—absolutely no bananas, broccoli, avocados, or dairy products of any kind this week! Week 2 is the Detox Anti-toxin Flush out Your Toxins Elimination Phase—absolutely no orange vegetables, soy products, rice, or pasta! And cut out all high-alkaline beverages and fruit!" Are you kidding me? Who makes these diets up? Where do these recommendations come from? All too often, they come from a smooth, charismatic personality with shaky or no credentials who is pulling the ideas out of thin air and exploiting our yearning for someone, anyone, who will give us a confident answer as to how we can lose weight. That's not what you want to base your health on. When was the last time you heard of anyone losing weight, getting healthier, and staying that way over the long term on a fad diet? I have yet to meet that person.

By definition, most diets set us up for failure. They have ridiculous, militaristic rules. They cut out food groups. They demonize wonderful, essential dietary elements like fats and carbohydrates—things that in moderation, your body needs, craves, and enjoys. Most diets are all too often based on bad science or laughably bogus nonscience.

Diets make us fear eating, hate certain foods, and torment ourselves with anxiety over falling off the wagon and spiraling into failure, desperate to hear about the next big diet. You could drive yourself completely crazy trying to keep track of all the latest alleged health and weight-loss breakthroughs that are reported in the media almost every single day—from acai and goji berries, to resveratrol, to this food or that pill reducing or increasing our risk of cancer. It's the media whipsaw effect: a study comes out, it's misreported in the media, another study comes out that contradicts the first one, and we all wind up confused.

Instead of jumping on a slickly advertised bandwagon, you need to find ways to ease yourself into a lifetime of healthy eating and physical activity over the long term. And one of the first steps is to give up on the idea that deprivation equals weight loss.

When it comes to food, Americans have a split personality. On the one hand, we're putting on weight at an alarming rate. Why? Well, there are many reasons:

- Portion sizes have exploded in recent years.

- The average American adult is consuming roughly 3,700 calories a day, when on average only about 2,000 to 2,800 is needed for a healthy weight, depending on our physical activity levels. That's right, we are consuming over 1,000 calories more per day than we should be!

- We are cooking less and eating much more food in restaurants that are serving us very unhealthy food, and where we are making the wrong food choices.

- We and our children are drinking increasingly huge amounts of sugary beverages.

- We are eating emotionally in response to stress and the pressures of daily life.

- We and our children are assaulted by billions of dollars' worth of marketing messages for unhealthy food.

- Most of us are not exercising nearly as much as we should be.

- We are bombarded with inaccurate, confusing, and bogus diet and nutrition information.

Yet on the other hand, at the same time many Americans are becoming so concerned with things like organic food, gluten, and "food toxins," that they run the risk of becoming overobsessed with healthy eating. As the *Washington Times* put it in 2008, "The line between eating healthfully and developing a full-blown eating disorder can be fuzzy for some people."

You don't need to stress out over every eating decision you and your family make. Your goal should be balance, moderation, and indulging in healthy food most of the time. In short, we need to learn to enjoy the things that are good for us.

How do you do that? Here's my strategy—whenever I sit down to eat, in the back of my mind I ask myself these four questions:

Dr. Stork's 4 Questions
That Lead to Savoring Food

- Is it delicious?
- Is it healthy?
- Will I feel good thirty minutes from now?
- Will a steady diet of this allow me to feel good in ten years?

I can't tell you how many times I've improved my food choices by thinking through these four ideas. Not only do the questions lead me to a healthier diet, but they keep me in a better mood—when I eat unhealthy food over the course of a few days, I can become grumpy and pessimistic. I feel like exercising less and instead end up parking my butt on the couch and roasting my eyeballs with rental movies until my head hurts.

The trouble is, many Americans have gotten used to the queasy, stoned, overwhelmed feeling you get after eating junk food. It has become a normal state, even a desired one because it becomes so natural to feel that way. It's time we rebooted our idea of deriving pleasure from food. Here's how to get started:

The 3 Paths to Food Pleasure

The Path	The Feeling	The Destination
Unhealthy Eating Patterns • Eating for a fast fix • Based on convenience • Regularly indulging in junk food and unhealthy foods	Fleeting pleasure, followed by semi-coma	Chronic disease, disability, depression, early death
Fad Diets • Short-term behaviors • Based on anecdotes, not evidence	Deprivation, fleeting pride in temporary small victories	Yo-yo weight fluctuations, disappointment
Healthy Eating Patterns • Eating to savor life • Allowing for treats • Based on evidence	Pleasure, followed by energy, power, stamina	Health, longevity, happiness

Let's call a halt to the junk food, fad diets, starving, fasting, detoxing, and silliness. The time has come for us to embrace a new way of indulging in delicious food every day to optimize our health.

ASK DR. STORK

Question: My co-worker says her nutritionist has worked wonders for her waistline and her health. She's urging me to go see him. It's a good idea to get health advice from a nutritionist, right?

Answer: It's a very good idea, as long as they've earned the credential "RD," which stands for "registered dietitian." This may come as a shock, but in most parts of the U.S., anyone can hang out a shingle and call themselves a nutritionist, a nutrition adviser, a holistic diet counselor, a registered dietary therapist, or any number of other official-sounding titles. But the titles are absolutely no assurance that the person has any true professional qualifications in the field of nutrition.

There's only one surefire way for you to identify a truly professionally certified expert who should be able to give you good nutrition advice, and that's to look for an RD. Registered dietitians are found in hospitals, HMO networks, community and public health settings, businesses, and private practice. They must meet a minimum of educational requirements and are certified by the American Dietetic Association, the nation's largest organization of food and nutrition professionals.

Note: Some RDs also call themselves nutritionists, because the public is more familiar with that term. Joy Bauer, RD, who appears on the *Today* show and is an excellent authority on nutrition, is an example. She refers to herself as a nutritionist, but most important, is a registered dietitian.

The Bottom Line: Many nutritionists are not registered dietitians, or RDs. Look for nutrition advisers with the RD credential.

Health Optimizer 2: Enjoy Healthy Eating Patterns

I admit, I used to be a total dummy when it came to nutrition. I know firsthand how easy it is to get caught up in the trap of unhealthy eating, because I grew up in an environment where unbalanced diets based on tons of meat with vegetables prepared in butter were the standard. That was just the dietary pattern—a big greasy breakfast of sausage, bacon, and ham flying off the griddle; a cheeseburger and fries for lunch; fried chicken or meat and potatoes for dinner.

In college I ate fast food almost every day, and I thought it was delicious and a perfectly normal lifestyle. I thought fried chicken was nutritious because it was chicken, and I thought anything labeled as "low fat," processed or otherwise, was good for me. After college, I focused on eating lower fat foods because that seemed all the rage, but I really had no idea what I was doing. I was lean, worked out regularly, and thought I was being really healthy.

But when I went to medical school, I realized I wasn't being healthy at all and that I needed to make a change.

For one thing, I had a great mentor who said to me, "Don't ever ask your patients to do something that you wouldn't do. If you ask them to eat fish, then you need to eat fish. If you ask them to cut out salt, you should cut out salt." I wanted to be a doctor who practiced what he preached, which meant I had to teach myself about nutrition. I know it sounds crazy, but unfortunately medical schools don't spend much time teaching about health and nutrition. They focus on disease instead.

But the biggest motivator to start eating healthier was the regular ordeal of working thirty-six hours straight in the hospital. I had to figure out how to keep awake and keep up my stamina.

I figured the one thing I could control during those thirty-plus hour stints was what I put in my body, so I began to make healthy meals to throw in my backpack. Instead of eating the hospital cafeteria food, I'd make a turkey sandwich with mustard and veggies on whole wheat. Instead of hitting up the vending machine for candy and salty snacks, I munched on healthy energy bars when there wasn't time to eat a proper meal. I made as many "healthy tweaks" as I could think of. It worked. I had good energy and a good mind-set and I was able to thrive in the high-pressure environment of the hospital, and ever since, in the world of the ER.

At the same time, I plunged into the medical research on healthy eating, which I've continued to do to this day. I've reviewed the results of many hundreds of the most intensive research studies of nutrition and optimal health, and I've come to the same conclusion that most of the greatest scientists, doctors, professors, and other researchers who study the field are coming to: that a predominately plant-based diet is the eating pattern that is best for optimal health.

Note that plant-based doesn't mean plant-only. It means that plant-based foods should be the stars of your healthy eating pattern. Research strongly suggests this is the most effective eating pattern for weight control, for longevity, and for reducing the risks of heart disease, type 2 diabetes, and other diseases, including cancer. Researchers at the American Institute for Cancer Research, for example, report that foods like vegetables, fruits, whole grains, and beans give your body a symphony of minerals, vitamins, fiber, and phytochemicals that can protect you against cancer—so they recommend that at least two-thirds of your plate should be usually filled with vegetables, fruit, whole grains, and beans.

America has some of the flat-out greatest food in the world. But our food culture—the way we prepare, balance, and eat that food—has thrown us over the cliff into an abyss where we are eating 1,000 calories a day more than we should, and eating a terribly unhealthy pattern of foods. Things have gotten so bad that, borrowing lessons from the antismoking campaign, we should probably post a health notice on every food package and at every restaurant, cafeteria, and store that sells food in America.

I suggest the following—feel free to quote me, FDA!

DR. STORK'S NATIONAL HEALTH WARNING

If over time you consume excessive calories, saturated fat, and sodium, and you don't enjoy regular physical activity, you are:

- Increasing your risk for premature death, time spent in the hospital, and wasting large amounts of money on avoidable medications and medical costs.
- Increasing your risk for both sudden death and years of severe disability.
- Increasing your risk of obesity, heart attack, stroke, cardiovascular disease, high blood pressure, metabolic syndrome, several forms of cancer, osteoarthritis, Alzheimer's disease, osteoporosis, and type 2 diabetes, the impact of the latter of which can include blindness, kidney failure, and the amputation of fingers, toes, hands, feet, and legs.
- Directly contributing to the collapse of the American health care system and helping create a nightmare crisis for our children and grandchildren.

The *good news* is: if over time you enjoy healthy eating patterns based largely on a wide variety of fruits and vegetables, whole grains, and healthy foods like fish, beans, nuts, and legumes, and you get regular physical activity, you are optimizing your health by reducing your risk of developing a very wide spectrum of chronic diseases.

It turns out that the best diet you can follow—which isn't really a diet at all—is whatever series of overall healthy eating patterns you can create for yourself that you can enjoy over the long term, through the course of your life. I urge you to become your own diet guru by learning the basics of optimal nutrition and then creating a healthy eating pattern that is designed just for you. In the following pages, I'll explain how, and the great news is this: it's surprisingly simple.

Notice I said simple—it's not necessarily easy. I know how hard it is for many people to eat healthy and stick with it, and how hard it can be to get to a healthy weight. But it absolutely is possible, and let me tell you, when you do it, the payoff is incredible, both in terms of your health and the way you feel. So how do you get started?

The first step toward developing a personal healthy pattern is to not overfocus on individual foods, or individual vitamins or ingredients, and not to follow the headlines toward one fad diet or a single promising vitamin study. Instead, think of the big picture by focusing on overall healthy patterns of eating. These healthy patterns are to be enjoyed over the long term and are not based on denial and cutting things out, but on savoring the joy of food, while keeping in mind some basic guidelines.

ASK DR. STORK

Question: Should I buy only organic food?

Answer: If you can afford the high prices, go for it! I like the idea of my food being grown without synthetic chemicals. But I'm also a cost-conscious consumer and I realize that organic is usually significantly more expensive than regular food, so an option is to cherry-pick the organic foods you buy.

The research on the health benefits of organic food is a mixed bag. Critics of conventional food production, such as the nonprofit Environmental Working Group, point to the purported toxic effects of pesticides, especially to babies and children, such as damage to the hormonal and nervous systems and increased cancer risk.

Other experts say there's no clear evidence that organic is healthier and that the important point is simply to get more people to eat fruits and veggies, period. In the end, buying organic is a personal choice. I tend to buy more organic foods than conventional, but if I can peel an item, like avocados, for instance, I often buy conventional. I also always thoroughly wash all my produce before I eat it, even including items that say "organic prewashed."

The Bottom Line: Consider buying organic versions of these "dirty dozen" produce items, which, according to a major analysis by the Environmental Working Group (EWG), are the highest in average tested pesticide content:

1. Peaches*
2. Apples*
3. Bell peppers*
4. Celery
5. Nectarines
6. Strawberries
7. Cherries
8. Kale
9. Lettuce
10. Grapes (imported)
11. Carrots
12. Pears

* Worst

And don't feel like you need to buy organic versions of "the clean fifteen" (the foods lowest in pesticides). The EWG's analysis ranked these items as being lowest in pesticides, so if cost is an issue for you, consider buying conventional versions of:

1. Onions*
2. Avocados*
3. Sweet corn*
4. Pineapples
5. Mangoes
6. Asparagus
7. Sweet peas
8. Kiwi
9. Cabbage
10. Eggplant
11. Papaya
12. Watermelon
13. Broccoli
14. Tomatoes
15. Sweet potatoes

* Best

Do you know what healthy eating approach is greatly admired and respected by the best, hard-core nutritional experts? It's not the Grapefruit Diet, the Cabbage Soup Diet, or any of the multitude of pills, shakes, or internet diet plans out there. In fact, it's not a fad diet at all—it's a dietary pattern called the Mediterranean diet.

The traditional Mediterranean diet is a pattern of eating based on the traditional diets of the people who live in the lands of the Mediterranean, especially Greece and Crete. The traditional Mediterranean diet pattern is considered close to a gold standard of optimal eating for health and longevity. Experts at the Department of Nutrition at the Harvard School of Public Health, for example, have studied the Mediterranean diet in great depth, and come to this extraordinary conclusion: "Together with regular physical activity and not smoking, our analyses suggest that over 80% of coronary heart disease, 70% of stroke, and 90% of type 2 diabetes can be avoided by healthy food choices that are consistent with the traditional Mediterranean diet."

How exactly does the Mediterranean diet's healthy eating pattern work to provide these benefits? The funny thing is we don't really know. Like any other healthy eating pattern, the Mediterranean diet seems to be a mysterious symphony that depends on the infinitely complex interactions between the thousands of players, rather than being driven by a few key components. Researchers used to think that perhaps the possible heart-protective powers of olive oil or red wine in the Mediterranean diet were key, but they are now most intrigued by the synergistic and "symphonic" effects of the overall pattern, which ironically can't be measured.

So what exactly is the Mediterranean dietary pattern, and how can you adopt its lessons in your life?

It's easiest to explain by using a food pyramid. Normally, I don't like the idea of food pyramids, because they can be confusing, they can seem restricting, and no one food pyramid fits all people. But this Mediterranean Diet Pyramid, introduced last year by the food think tank Oldways Preservation Trust, comes close to being perfect.* This one diagram cuts through the infinity of bad nutritional information clutter out there and synthesizes everything down to a pattern everyone can understand.

I think this chart should be taped to every kitchen refrigerator in America. For that matter, it should be taped to the wall of every primary care doctor and family doctor's office as a poster and given as a handout every time they see a patient. It should be hung in a position of prominence in every school and hospital in America.

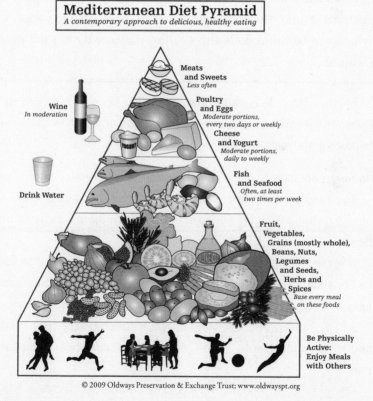

Mediterranean Diet Pyramid
A contemporary approach to delicious, healthy eating

Meats
and Sweets
Less often

Wine
In moderation

Poultry
and Eggs
*Moderate portions,
every two days or weekly*

Cheese
and Yogurt
*Moderate portions,
daily to weekly*

Fish
and Seafood
*Often, at least
two times per week*

Drink Water

Fruit,
Vegetables,
Grains (mostly whole),
Beans, Nuts,
Legumes
and Seeds,
Herbs and
Spices
*Base every meal
on these foods*

Be Physically
Active:
Enjoy Meals
with Others

---

* The only thing I would add to this chart is that if you enjoy meat and poultry, make them lean choices in sensible portions, and if you enjoy dairy products, choose low-fat options. Also, see my important note on alcohol on page 42.

Remember, this is not a fad diet with hard-and-fast rules to follow. It is an example of a healthy pattern to inspire you to start thinking about nutritious, delicious eating. Living in Tennessee much of the time, I rarely get to eat actual authentic Mediterranean food, but I subconsciously follow many of the food patterns shown in the chart—like piling on the whole grains, fruits and veggies, herbs and spices, and of course, engaging in physical activity!

Look closely at the pyramid. Note that meats and sweets are allowed—just remember to eat them less often. Notice how fish dominates the chart much more than meat—that's how your eating pattern should be. See how it allows for near-infinite variety and for you to enjoy multiple healthy eating patterns within the overall guidelines?

ASK DR. STORK

Question: Should I be drinking a glass or two of red wine each day to protect my heart?

Answer: I absolutely love a good glass of red wine with dinner.

If you enjoy moderate amounts of alcohol responsibly and don't have a history of alcohol abuse or dependency, there may be some benefit.

One theory is that that red wine can protect against heart disease by boosting, to a small extent, "good" HDL cholesterol, plus possibly offering an anticlotting benefit, perhaps from the substance known as resveratrol. Speculation has focused on the flavonoids and other antioxidants in red wine as reducing heart disease risk.

Many studies seem to associate moderate alcohol consumption (two drinks a day for men, one for women*) with the above-mentioned heart benefits and possible protection against

Alzheimer's disease. It is important to note these are only observational studies comparing sample populations, not actual trials that put the theory to the test.

What about the famous "French paradox"? France has a diet high in meat, cheese, and butter, but has lower heart disease mortality than the U.S. and an additional year of overall life expectancy. This paradox is often ascribed to the supposed health benefits of red wine. But the French have traditionally consumed several hundred fewer calories per day on average than Americans and eat less saturated fat overall. The French also get more physical activity in their daily lives than Americans do, according to experts at the University of California-Berkeley, who conclude that "It would be unwise to conclude from all this that drinking wine will make up for a diet high in calories and saturated fat," like the typical American diet.

According to the American Heart Association (AHA), there is no scientific proof that drinking wine or any alcoholic beverage can replace the effective strategies of controlling your weight, lowering your cholesterol and blood pressure, getting enough physical activity, and following a healthy diet, all of which reduce your risk for heart disease. "How alcohol or wine affects cardiovascular risk merits further research," says the AHA, "but right now the (AHA) does not recommend drinking wine or any other form of alcohol to gain these potential benefits."

As an ER doctor, I also see the ravaging effects of alcohol, in the form of alcoholism, drunk driving, and other life-threatening problems. The dangers of alcohol abuse are legion, and well known: 12,000 people are killed in drunk driving accidents yearly, and the social devastation linked to alcoholism, including domestic violence and child abuse, is tragic. Excessive alcohol consumption is also a risk factor tied to increased risks of breast cancer and several other cancers, stroke, liver disease, workplace and firearms injuries, high blood pressure, and suicide.

The Bottom Line: If you drink alcohol, do so in moderation. That means one or two drinks per day for men and one drink per day for women.*

It's impossible to predict in which people alcoholism will become a problem. Given these and other risks, the American Heart Association cautions people not to start drinking if they do not already drink alcohol. And pregnant women shouldn't drink alcohol in any form. It can harm the baby, including causing birth defects.

* A drink is one 12 oz. beer, 4 oz. of wine, 1.5 oz. of 80-proof spirits, or 1 oz. of 100-proof spirits.

There are no added sugars on the pyramid, except for the allowance of a little dessert on top, to be enjoyed "less often." There's no sweetened soda, diet soda, or vitamin and sugar-enhanced water. That stuff contains empty calories, the food equivalent of a total waste of money. It is of no benefit to your health, and in some cases it's damaging to it. If you enjoy one every now and then, don't worry about it, but remember, moderation is the key! There are no processed junk foods like chips, French fries, cheese balls, or toaster pastries. They, too, are mostly empty calories, so eat them sparingly. Also, there's no added salt, since too much sodium can elevate your blood pressure. Flavor your food with herbs and spices instead. And there are no vitamin pills or other supplements, which, with a few exceptions, are largely unproven to be effective.

The Bottom Line: You should enjoy American food, Mexican food, Thai food, Japanese food, Chinese food, Mediterranean food, any and all kinds of food you like, as long as you remember to prepare them in a healthy way while building your overall eating patterns largely on foods like fruits, veggies, whole grains, fish, beans, nuts, and legumes.

There is no single diet or exact combination of foods that is best for everyone and no pyramid that's perfect for everyone. Depending on where you live, your culture, and the size of your bank account, you should create your very own food pyramid to suit your tastes and budget. I encourage you to make a list of healthy and nutritious foods that you enjoy that fit into each category of the Mediterranean diet, keeping the pyramid's proportions in mind, and go buy them at the grocery store. You choose what to put on your list. Fill the pyramid—and your grocery cart—with the things you love. While your exact healthy eating pattern will be different from everyone else's, based on your tastes, these are general guideposts, based on the best, latest nutritional research, that will navigate you toward the optimal pattern you can design yourself.

Dr. Stork's 7 Guidelines for Designing Your Optimal Healthy Eating Patterns (or How to Build Your Perfect Anti-Diet)

1. Base your eating patterns largely on "whole plants"—whole fruits, whole vegetables, and whole grains.

2. Embrace sources of "good" fats (like fish, olive oil, and nuts), "good" carbs (like whole grains), and lean protein (like beans, legumes, and, if you eat meat or poultry, lean cuts).

3. Base your eating on true pleasure. Enjoy the most delicious, healthy foods over the long term, while allowing for balance, moderation, variety, and indulgences.

4. Be inspired by the healthy eating patterns that are backed up by good evidence—like the traditional diets of the Mediterranean.

5. Make regular physical activity part of your lifestyle—think of sneakers as an essential food group.

6. Be consistent. Your healthy eating patterns should not be cycled in and out, they should be enjoyed over the long term.

7. Consult an expert. Optimal healthy eating patterns are best established with the help of a doctor or registered dietitian.

Health Optimizer 3: Enjoy Many Different Kinds of Whole Veggies and Fruit

Before I begin to preach to you about the joys of a fruit and vegetable-rich lifestyle, I have to admit that there are days when I absolutely don't eat my five to ten servings of fruit and veggies. Some days I'm lucky if the thought of a leafy green or an orange even crosses my mind.

I have a friend who grows, and eats, all his own fruits and vegetables. I wish I could be like him. But when I get home after twelve hours on my feet I'm usually in no mood to whip up a dinner of salmon and veggies from scratch.

The majority of the time, however, I do manage to find the time to load up on the produce. My overall eating pattern is very healthy, and I make it as easy on myself as possible by taking shortcuts. I am proof positive that you can eat healthy with minimal effort and time. How?

I'll take two minutes in the morning to throw a bunch of frozen fruit in the blender, toss in some whey protein powder and low fat Greek yogurt, and whip up a fantastic, filling smoothie. I'll have a veggie burger for lunch on whole wheat with tomatoes, avocados, and whatever other veggies I have on hand. On busy days, my meals don't take long to prepare, they aren't expensive, and they taste great, and it's certainly not because I'm some great cook—it all starts with what I buy at the grocery store.

The best thing you can start doing today that will get you on your way to optimizing your health through food is to go to the supermarket, walk to the produce section, and stand there and admire the beautiful shapes, gorgeous colors, and magnificent variety that stretches out before you in the form of whole fruits and vegetables.

As you stand there, close your eyes and make yourself a promise. Resolve that from that moment on, *this* is where you're going to spend more of your time shopping. Realize this is a key to your good health, and the heart of your new food life, a new life of eating to truly savor food. Decide that from now on you're going to enjoy many different kinds of whole veggies and fruit.

I am not rational on the subject of fruit and vegetables. I am crazy about them. I stuff veggies into my sandwiches, stir-fries, and pasta dinners. I consider fruit and veggies the bedrock of my healthy, delicious eating patterns. I know you've heard it before—I'm hardly the first person to go around saying "eat more fruits and vegetables." But it is crucial that you understand one simple fact that can totally change your life: one of the greatest things you will ever do for your health is to make the commitment to build your eating patterns upon a wide variety of many fruits and vegetables. *So learn to enjoy them!*

I know for some people, the idea of enjoying fruits and vegetables may seem like a stretch. You might be thinking, "Nice idea, Travis, but forget it. I hate vegetables, always have, always will, and nothing you tell me will ever get me to eat them except occasionally and under protest."

This is what I have to say to you: you've been brainwashed by our unhealthy food culture to think this way. The food companies and restaurant companies have reprogrammed your body's natural biology to crave excessively processed foods, saturated fat, sugar, and sodium—when what it really craves is a wide variety of fruits and vegetables and other superpowerful foods.

Tragically, the share of Americans forty to seventy-four years old who consume a minimum of five fruits and vegetables a day has plunged from 42 percent to 26 percent in the last twenty years.

This is the point in the book when I whip out a megaphone and stand on a soapbox. Here's my junk-food speech. Can I have a drum-roll, please?

DR. STORK'S JUNK-FOOD SPEECH

Just because everyone else in your neighborhood has kitchens full of soda pop, white bread, potato chips, processed cheese, mayo, pastries, high fat and sodium frozen dinners, and tubs of ice cream the size of water buckets, that's absolutely no reason you should, too.

There's nothing intrinsically evil about any of these foods in and of themselves, if you enjoy modest portions of them occasionally. But when they are the basis of your eating patterns, you are in for some big-time health trouble.

You and your family need to know that a high-calorie, low-nutrient eating pattern of too much added sugar, sodium, saturated fat, and processed foods will, over time, make you sick and may even kill you. You must realize that this is a biologically abnormal, and medically dangerous, lifestyle for you to have.

Make your home a mostly junk-food-free zone.

You may be addicted to the false feeling of satisfaction that these kinds of foods—which, let's face it, have become staples in many Americans' lives—can give you. But you are much stronger and more powerful than you think. You can break the spell. And when you do, the payoff will be spectacular—trust me.

I had my own doubts about whether I could enjoy a mostly junk-food-free lifestyle until I actually started sampling how many different mouthwatering, super-filling fruits and veggies the Earth has to offer.

In the produce section of any halfway decent supermarket in America, you'll probably find at least one hundred fruit and vegetable choices in the produce section, plus lots more in the canned and frozen foods sections. They're all good, as long as they don't have sugar or sodium added to them. Don't buy into the myths put forward by some self-appointed health gurus that this fruit or that veggie is bad for you and should be avoided. If you crack open the average health and diet book, you can find all kinds of outrageous, totally inaccurate slander being cast upon certain produce items, such as, "No bananas in Week 1—they are pure sugar and you need to eliminate your sugar cravings to shock your system in this induction phase of the diet!" Or, "Absolutely no avocados! They are high alkaline and will unbalance your hormones." This is pure baloney. It is usually based on a health guru pulling a bad idea out of thin air, or incorrectly extrapolating a conclusion from a thin line of research.

ASK DR. STORK

Question: What vegetable and fruit "superfoods" do you recommend?

Answer: I recommend them all. It's really not accurate to elevate a few fruits or veggies far above the others in terms of nutrition. They are all fantastic. "Superfoods" is a misnomer, and I'm reluctant to use the phrase.

It is tempting to join the stampede toward one berry or another because of a single study that appears to show benefits, or a lab experiment that suggests disease-fighting potential with this antioxidant or that phytonutrient. But you can't stake your health on little pieces of the puzzle—instead, keep focused on the big picture. The research and the science tell us that the real superfood is the combination of many different fruits and veggies.

Having said that, there are certain categories of fruit and veggies that are so nutritious that they deserve special mention as elite players you should remember to rotate into your healthy eating patterns: berries; leafy greens; cruciferous veggies like broccoli, Brussels sprouts, cabbage, and kale; sweet potatoes; avocados; Concord grapes; and legumes like peas, beans, and lentils.

Beans are so good they occupy a special category of nutrition for me. They contain fiber, lots of protein (rare for a plant-based food), antioxidants, and are extremely convenient and cheap. You can enjoy them as an affordable, versatile, no-fat, no-cholesterol meat substitute, or to complement any main dish as well as soups and salads. If you enjoy beans, they should be a regular star of your food lifestyle, as they are, for example, in the Mediterranean diet.

You can develop your own personalized list of superfoods simply by going to the produce section and filling up a shopping basket with samples of your five favorite fruits and veggies, plus two or three you've never tried before. Now, that's a basket of superfood—they're all great!

The Bottom Line: All fruits and vegetables are superfoods, when you eat lots of different kinds, all the time.

Whenever you hear a health guru criticize a particular whole fruit or vegetable, you should run fast in the opposite direction. As long as you eat lots of different veggies and fruit, usually in their whole and unprocessed forms (for example, smoothies are fine, in fact, they're fantastic, as long as you don't add extra sugars), you are optimizing your health.

One possible exception is the white potato, which some experts legitimately argue should be considered inferior because it is a high "glycemic index" food that can spike your blood sugar, too much of which could theoretically lead to weight gain. Personally, I believe potatoes are a filling, tasty, and nutritious veggie to rotate into your life along with scores of others, but sweet potatoes or yams pack a bigger health punch than white potatoes, from extra nutrients to slower-burning carbohydrates.

Exactly how do fruits and veggies optimize our health? There are many good theories, but no one has cracked the scientific code yet. Maybe they reduce inflammation and oxidative stress that promote chronic disease. Maybe they inhibit the activation of cancerous tumors. Maybe they help us achieve a healthy body weight by making us feel full on fewer calories, ultimately displacing less healthy foods from our diet.

Once again, it seems to be the "synergistic" effect of the thousands and thousands of ingredients in different fruits and veggies working together in a beautiful, and as-yet mysterious symphony. The ingredients include vitamins, minerals, antioxidants, fiber, flavonoids, carotenoids such as lycopene, phenolics, alkaloids, nitrogen-containing compounds, organosulfur compounds, polyphelols, plant sterols, other plant compounds like resveratrol, and probably hundreds of things we don't even know about yet. One thing is becoming increasingly clear: the foods that grow from the ground have fantastic health benefits.

Here are just a few of the specific health benefits of fruit and veggies, and examples of where to get them, according to www.my pyramid.gov:

Fiber

Diets rich in fiber have been shown to have a number of benefits, including decreased risk of coronary artery disease.

Good fruit and vegetable sources: Navy beans, kidney beans, black beans, pinto beans, lima beans, white beans, soybeans, split peas, chickpeas, black-eyed peas, lentils, artichokes, pears, raspberries, blackberries, prunes, figs, dates, bananas, oranges.

Folate*

Healthful diets with adequate folate may reduce a woman's risk of having a child with a brain or spinal cord defect.

Good fruit and vegetable sources: Black-eyed peas, cooked spinach, great northern beans, asparagus, citrus fruits.

Potassium

Diets rich in potassium may help to maintain a healthy blood pressure.

Good fruit and vegetable sources: Sweet potatoes, tomato paste, bananas, tomato puree, white potatoes, white beans, lima beans, cooked greens, carrot juice, prune juice.

Vitamin A

Vitamin A keeps eyes and skin healthy and helps to protect against infections.

Good fruit and vegetable sources: Sweet potatoes, pumpkin, carrots, spinach, turnip greens, mustard greens, kale, collard greens, winter squash, cantaloupe, red peppers, Chinese cabbage.

Vitamin C

Vitamin C is important for the growth of all body tissue, and it helps heal cuts and wounds and keep teeth and gums healthy.

---

* The Institute of Medicine recommends that women of childbearing age who may become pregnant consume 400 micrograms of synthetic folic acid per day to supplement the folate they receive from a varied diet. Synthetic folic acid can be obtained from eating fortified foods or taking a supplement.

Good fruit and vegetable sources: Red and green peppers, kiwi, strawberries, sweet potatoes, kale, cantaloupe, broccoli, pineapple, Brussels sprouts, oranges, mangoes, tomato juice, cauliflower.

ASK DR. STORK

Question: Is it healthy to follow a vegetarian diet?

Answer: A vegetarian diet can absolutely be a healthy one and can meet all your requirements for nutrients if you make sure to cover all your nutritional bases. The key is to consume a variety of foods and the proper quantity of foods to meet your calorie requirements. Compared to an eating pattern rich in red meat, the benefits of a balanced vegetarian diet can include less saturated fat, more complex carbohydrates, more fiber, and more phytochemicals and other plant nutrients.

Nutrients that vegetarians need to be sure to get enough of include protein, iron, calcium, zinc, and vitamin B_{12}. Here's a rundown on how to get those nutrients, plus other vegetarian tips, all from the mypyramid.gov website, which is filled with good information on this and many other healthy eating topics:

- **Protein** has many important functions in the body and is essential for growth and maintenance. Protein needs can easily be met by eating a variety of plant-based foods. (Combining different protein sources in the same meal is not necessary.) Sources of protein for vegetarians include beans, nuts, nut butters, peas, and soy products (tofu, tempeh, veggie burgers). Milk products and eggs are also good protein sources for lacto-ovo vegetarians.
- **Iron** functions primarily as a carrier of oxygen in the blood. Iron sources for vegetarians include iron-fortified breakfast cereals, spinach, kidney beans, black-eyed peas, lentils, turnip greens,

molasses, whole wheat breads, peas, and some dried fruits (dried apricots, prunes, raisins).

- **Calcium** is used for building bones and teeth and in maintaining bone strength. Sources of calcium for vegetarians include fortified breakfast cereals, soy products (tofu, soy-based beverages), calcium-fortified orange juice, and some dark green leafy vegetables (collard greens, turnip greens, bok choy, mustard greens). Milk products are excellent calcium sources for lacto-vegetarians.
- **Zinc** is necessary for many biochemical reactions and also helps the immune system function properly. Sources of zinc for vegetarians include many types of beans (white beans, kidney beans, and chickpeas), zinc-fortified breakfast cereals, wheat germ, and pumpkin seeds. Milk products are a zinc source for lacto-vegetarians.
- **Vitamin B$_{12}$** is found in animal products and some fortified foods. Sources of vitamin B$_{12}$ for vegetarians include milk products, eggs, and foods that have been fortified with vitamin B$_{12}$. These include some breakfast cereals, soy-based beverages, veggie burgers, and nutritional yeast.

The Bottom Line: If you want to go vegetarian, go for it! Just remember to cover your nutritional bases, and as you plan your food choices, it's a great idea to consult with a registered dietitian and your doctor.

Health Optimizer 4: Switch in the Whole Grains

Every time you reach for a piece of bread, a plate of pasta, or a bowl of cereal, you have an opportunity to eat to savor life and optimize your health by choosing the whole grain option. I max up on whole grains every chance I get, by choosing foods like whole grain oatmeal snacks, whole wheat pasta, and whole wheat bread.

A whole grain is exactly that—a grain product that contains all three parts of the grain kernel: the bran, germ, and endosperm. A refined grain product like white bread, by contrast, has had the bran and germ stripped out, removing much of the nutrients, although a little bit gets added back in when it is "enriched" by the manufacturer.

According to the 2005 U.S. Dietary Guidelines for Americans, children should be eating at least two to three servings of whole grains per day, and adults should have at least three to five servings, but the average American eats less than one serving a day, and 40 percent of us don't eat any whole grains at all. Clearly we need to improve those stats.

Why? Here are four great reasons, according to the Dietary Guidelines for Americans:

How Whole Grains Help Optimize Your Health

- Whole grains are a key source of complex carbohydrates, or "good" carbs, which your body needs for everyday energy. Like fruits and vegetables, whole grains contain health-promoting nutrients like antioxidants, B vitamins, vitamin E, magnesium, selenium, iron, and fiber.

- Eating patterns rich in whole grains may reduce the risks of heart disease, stroke, cancer, diabetes, and obesity.

- People who regularly eat whole grains have a lower risk of obesity, as measured by their body mass index and waist-to-hip ratios. They also have lower cholesterol levels.

- Whole grains are an important source of fiber. Consuming foods rich in fiber, like whole grains, as part of a healthy diet, reduces the risk of coronary heart disease. Fiber is also important for proper bowel function. It helps reduce constipation and diverticulosis. In addition, fiber-containing foods such as whole grains help provide a feeling of fullness with fewer calories.

Examples of whole grain foods, when they include the endosperm, germ, and bran, are: whole wheat, oats and oatmeal, brown rice, rye, barley, corn (including whole cornmeal and popcorn), and buckwheat. There are more exotic whole grains as well, many of which you may not have tried, but might want to check out, such as: colored rice, wild rice, amaranth, kasha, millet, bulgur, quinoa, and sorghum.

Tips for Savoring Whole Grains

Breakfast: Switch out your overly refined breakfast cereals and go for whole grain options like oatmeal. Read the back of the cereal package and make sure the first ingredient listed is one of the whole grains listed above. Instead of white-flour-based waffles, muffins, and pancakes, get the whole grain versions.

Lunch: Switch out your white bread for whole grain bread. I do this every single day.

Dinner: Get a rice cooker and make brown rice a regular feature at your dinner table, or zap up some plain microwavable brown rice. Try whole wheat pasta—and give yourself time to learn to appreciate its heartier taste and thicker texture. Many restaurants now offer brown rice and whole wheat pasta, so always ask if you can substitute!

Beware!

Here are some tips for getting the most out of your whole grains:

- Some food companies use marketing tricks to fool us into thinking a product is whole grain when it isn't. The words "multigrain," "12 grain," "hearty grains," "stone ground," "mixed grains," and "made with whole grains" are no guarantee that the product is 100 percent whole grain or even mostly whole grain.

• To make sure you're getting a whole grain product, check the ingredient list. A whole grain should be the first ingredient listed. For instance, the first ingredient should say "whole wheat," not "cracked wheat," "wheat," "wheat flour," or any other variation on a theme other than the word "whole."

ASK DR. STORK

Question: What do you think of gluten-free diets?

Answer: I had a gluten-free slice of banana bread recently and it tasted great.

I'm not gluten intolerant, it just happened to be there for the taking and I enjoyed it.

Gluten-free food has become a health craze, and many people are jumping on the bandwagon, including companies that are now selling a multitude of food products that trumpet the fact that they contain no gluten.

Gluten is a protein found in wheat, barley, and rye. It is found widely throughout the food system, especially in ubiquitous foods like pasta and bread, and it's not always listed on food labels. People with celiac disease are allergic to gluten, and when they consume it, their small intestine is damaged and nutrients get poorly absorbed, triggering a number of symptoms. Approximately two to three million Americans have celiac disease, and unfortunately many don't even realize they have it. The only effective treatment is to cut out all gluten in the diet.

In my medical practice, I am noticing more and more people being diagnosed with celiac disease, which may be a positive outgrowth of greater awareness of the problem. For these people, the rise in gluten-free food is a terrific thing.

Some people, however, are blaming gluten for a host of other medical problems. They believe that even for people who don't have celiac disease, a gluten-free diet can help people lose weight, gain energy and focus, and mitigate symptoms of conditions like fibromyalgia, attention deficit/hyperactivity disorder (ADHD), and autism.

While probably little harm can come from following a gluten-free diet (other than the damage to your pocketbook from the premium prices of many gluten-free foods), I have not seen convincing medical evidence of any these claims.

The Bottom Line: If you have persistent, unexplained gastrointestinal symptoms like pain, vomiting, constipation, diarrhea, poor weight gain, or unexplained weight loss, you may be allergic to gluten. Talk with your doctor. There are simple tests for gluten sensitivity, so if you're concerned that you might be affected, ask your doctor about getting tested. However, if you have not been medically diagnosed with celiac disease or a gluten sensitivity, there's no reason for you to be on a gluten-free diet.

Health Optimizer 5: Enjoy More Fish

It's true-confessions time again: I am not very good at preparing fish. I grew up in a fish-poor food culture, and until I hit my thirties it rarely occurred to me to eat it more than once a month or so. When I was growing up, my family was busy broiling steaks and grilling chicken breasts—we never really figured out how to prepare fish.

There are still weeks when I'll go without eating fish, but now I'll get mad at myself, because I know better.

Outside of tuna fish sandwiches, fish is still a bit player in the lives of many Americans, which is a real shame because it's so good for us.

A big component of the Eat to Savor Life Plan is to include fish as a regular part of your diet. Seafood, and especially "fatty fish" like salmon, trout, and sardines, is a nutritional superstar for many reasons:

- Fish is rich in high-quality protein, iron, B vitamins, and other nutrients like potassium, phosphorous, and selenium.

- Fish is relatively low in saturated fat and is a good replacement for meat that may be high in saturated fat.

- Fatty fish is rich in "good" polyunsaturated fats, and particularly the omega-3 fatty acids eicosapentaenoic acid (EPA) and docosapentaenoic acid (DHA). Some plant-based foods, like flaxseed and walnuts, also contain omega-3 fatty acids, and are therefore great to have in your diet. Fish oil supplements are also a good source of omega-3s. I take one every morning, as I admit I don't always eat as much fish as I'd like during the week.

- Omega-3 fatty acids may be protective against cardiovascular disease and heart attacks by lowering triglyceride and cholesterol levels, relaxing blood vessels, decreasing blood pressure, modulating electrical activity in the heart, and making blood less sticky. So far, the strongest benefit appears to be protection against death from heart attacks.

- Babies whose mothers consume EPA and DHA when pregnant may enjoy better vision, growth, and brain development. In 2004, the Food and Drug Administration advised that "women and young children in particular should include fish or shellfish in their diets due to the many nutritional benefits."

- Researchers are studying whether omega-3 fatty acids may play a role in countering depression and other mental health problems.

It's important to note that most of the research on omega-3s, both in fish and from supplements, is not based on randomized clinical trials, meaning it is speculative and needs to be confirmed. The research is so promising, however, that the American Heart Association has issued guidelines encouraging us to eat fish to reap the benefits of omega-3s:

Population: Patients without documented coronary heart disease (CHD)	Recommendation: Eat a variety of (preferably fatty) fish at least twice a week. Include oils and foods rich in alpha-linolenic acid (flaxseed, canola, and soybean oils; flaxseed and walnuts).
Population: Patients with documented CHD	Recommendation: Consume about 1 gram of EPA+DHA per day, preferably from fatty fish. EPA+DHA in capsule form could be considered in consultation with the physician.
Population: Patients who need to lower triglycerides (see page 129 for more on triglycerides).	Recommendation: 2 to 4 grams of EPA+DHA per day provided as capsules under a physician's care.

There are a few cautions when it comes to fish oils. According to experts at the University of California—Berkeley, "The decreased ability of your blood to clot has a negative side, notably an increased risk of hemorrhagic stroke. People with bleeding disorders, those taking anticoagulants, or those with uncontrolled hypertension (who are already at high risk for a stroke) should definitely not take fish oil capsules." High doses of fish oil, they add, can suppress certain aspects of the immune system. Bottom line: consult your doctor before taking fish oil supplements.

There are also cautions regarding fish and mercury consumption for women who might become pregnant, women who are pregnant, nursing mothers, and young children, so talk to your doctor if the situation is appropriate to you. Also, if you eat an especially large amount of fish in your diet and are concerned about mercury poisoning, which can cause nonspecific neurologic symptoms, I also strongly advise you to discuss this with your doctor.

Not all fish are created equal when it comes to consumption. Some types have high concentrations of mercury or other pollutants, and some are harvested in ways that are eco-unfriendly, or not sustainable. There is no simple rule of thumb for choosing fish—some salmon is good, some is less good; some farmed fish is good, some is less so. Luckily, the folks at the Environmental Defense Fund have done a lot of homework for us, and they've come up with these two handy charts we can use to help guide our fish choices—a Pocket Seafood Selector and a Pocket Sushi Selector.

The charts highlight good and bad options, as ranked by the health impact on the oceans and on health, and as measured by the presence of beneficial omega-3s. The charts, and more details on specific fish, are also available in color as a free download at the sites indicated below.

For more details on specific types of fish, visit www.edf.org and search for "seafood selector."

Seafood Selector

Fish Choices That Are Good for You and the Ocean

The same kind of fish may appear on more than one list of choices, depending on where it comes from, whether it was caught or farmed, and the type of fishing gear used. To learn more about choosing ocean-friendly fish, visit www.edf.org/seafood.

Best Choices	OK Choices	Worst Choices
Abalone (farmed)	Basa/swai/tra	Caviar/sturgeon
Barramundi (U.S.)	Caviar/sturgeon	(imported wild)
Catfish (U.S.)	(farmed)	†Chilean seabass
*Char, Arctic (farmed)	Clams (wild)	Cod, Atlantic
Clams (farmed)	Cod, Pacific (trawl)	Crab, king (imported)
Clams, softshell	†Crab, blue	Crawfish (China)
Cod, Pacific (bottom	Crab, king (U.S.)	Flounder/sole (Atlantic)
longline)	Crab, snow/tanner	†Grouper
Crab, Dungeness	Flounder/sole (Pacific)	Haddock (trawl)
Crab, stone	Haddock (hook-and-line)	Halibut, Atlantic
Crawfish (U.S.)	*Herring, Atlantic	Mahimahi (imported
Halibut, Pacific	Lobster, American/	longline)
Lobster, spiny (U.S.)	Maine	Monkfish
*Mackerel, Atlantic	Lobster, spiny	†Orange roughy
Mahimahi (U.S. pole/	(Bahamas)	†Rockfish (Pacific trawl)
troll)	Mahimahi (U.S.	†Salmon, farmed or
Mullet (U.S.)	longline)	Atlantic
*Mussels (farmed)	*Oysters (wild)	†Shark
*Oysters (farmed)	Pollock, Alaska	Shrimp/prawns
*Sablefish/black cod	*Sablefish/black cod	(imported)
(Alaska, Canada)	(CA, OR, WA)	Skate
*Salmon (Alaska wild)	†Salmon (Washington	Snapper, red or
*Salmon, canned pink/	wild)	imported
sockeye	Scallops, sea	†Swordfish (imported)
*Sardines (U.S.)	(Canada, U.S.)	Tilapia (Asia)
Scallops, bay (farmed)	*Shrimp (U.S. wild)	†Tuna, bigeye (longline)
*Shrimp, pink (Oregon)	*Shrimp, northern	†Tuna, yellowfin
*Shrimp (U.S. farmed)	(Canada, U.S.)	(imported longline)
*Spot prawn (Canada)	Squid (except U.S.	†Tuna, bluefin
Squid, longfin (U.S.)	longfin)	
Striped bass (farmed)	†Swordfish (U.S.)	
Tilapia (U.S.)	Tilapia (Latin America)	
*Trout, rainbow (farmed)	†Tuna, yellowfin (U.S.	
*Tuna, albacore	longline)	
(Canada, U.S.)	Tuna, canned light	
Tuna, skipjack (pole/	†Tuna, canned white/	
troll)	albacore	
Wreckfish		

* Fish that are both good sources of heart-healthy omega-3s and low in contaminants.

† Fish high in mercury or PCBs.

© 2010 Environmental Defense Fund

Sushi Selector

Sushi Choices That Are Good for You and the Ocean

Sushi names: Fish are listed by their Japanese name, then English common name. Japanese names often refer to several types of fish, or to a specific cut of fish, and may appear in more than one category.

Raw fish: Sushi is often uncooked, and may contain parasites or microorganisms that cause food-borne illness. Pregnant women, young children, older adults, and people with immune conditions should not eat raw or partially cooked seafood. Freezing raw fish before preparing sushi significantly reduces, but does not eliminate, health risks.

Choosing fish: Sushi is rarely labeled with species names, where the fish came from, or whether it was caught or farmed. Ask your server, chef, or sushi purveyor for this information.

For more information, visit www.edf.org/seafood

Best Choices	OK Choices	Worst Choices
*Amaebi/Spot prawns (Canada)	*Amaebi/Spot prawns (U.S.)	Ankimo/Monkfish liver
Awabi/Abalone (U.S. farmed)	*Ebi/Shrimp (U.S. wild)	Ankoh/Monkfish
*Gindara/Sablefish (Alaska, Canada)	Gindara/Sablefish (CA, OR, WA)	Ebi/Shrimp (imported)
Hirame/Pacific halibut	Hamachi/Yellowtail (U.S.)	Hamachi/Yellowtail (Australia, Japan)
Hotate/Bay scallops (farmed)	Hirame/Flounders and soles (Pacific)	Hirame/Flounders and soles (Atlantic)
Ikura/Salmon roe (Alaska wild)	Hotate/Sea scallops (Canada, U.S.)	Hirame/Halibut (Atlantic)
*Iwana/Arctic char (farmed)	Ika/Squid	†Hon Maguro/Bluefin tuna
*Iwashi/Sardines (U.S.)	*Kaki/Oysters (wild)	Ikura/Salmon roe (farmed or Atlantic)
Izumidai/Tilapia (U.S.)	†Kani/Blue crab	Kani/King crab (imported)
*Kaki/Oysters (farmed)	Kani/King crab (U.S.)	†Maguro/Bigeye or yellowfin tuna (longline)
Masago/Smelt roe (Iceland)	Kani/Snow crab	†Sake/Salmon (farmed or Atlantic)
Mirugai/Geoduck, giant clam (wild)	Kanikama, Surimi/Alaska pollock	†Shiro Maguro/Albacore tuna (imported longline)
*Muurugai/Mussels (farmed)	Maguro/Bigeye or yellowfin tuna (pole/troll)	Tai/Red snapper
*Sake/Salmon (Alaska wild)	Masago/Smelt roe (Canada)	Tako/Octopus
Shiro Maguro/Albacore tuna (Canada, U.S.)	†Sake/Salmon (Washington wild)	†Toro/Bigeye or yellowfin tuna belly (longline)
Suzuki/Striped bass (farmed)	Tai/Red porgy (U.S.)	†Toro/Bluefin tuna belly
Uni/Sea urchin roe (Canada)	Toro/Bigeye or yellowfin tuna belly (pole/troll)	Unagi/Freshwater eel
	Uni/Sea urchin roe (California)	Uni/Sea urchin roe (Maine)

* Fish that are both good sources of heart-healthy omega-3s and low in contaminants.

† Fish high in mercury or PCBs.

© 2010 Environmental Defense Fund

Dr. Stork's Top Fish Tips

Here are some great fish choices for you to include in your Eat to Savor Life shopping list. According to the Environmental Defense Fund, they are both good sources of heart-healthy omega-3s and low in contaminants:

- Alaska salmon (all kinds)

- Arctic char (farmed)

- Atlantic mackerel

- Oysters (farmed)

- Sablefish/black cod (Alaska and Canada)

- Sardines (U.S.)

- Rainbow trout (farmed)

- Albacore tuna (U.S., and not the widely available canned varieties but more premium-priced, low-mercury canned products from eco-friendly, sustainable U.S. fisheries in the Pacific—brands include Wild Planet and EcoFish. Look for "albacore" and "U.S." on the package.)

Alaska salmon is a great choice for health and convenience. There are five types of Alaska salmon: pink, keta, sockeye, coho, and king salmon. They are all wild-caught, sustainably harvested, and eco-friendly. They're rich in omega-3s and very low in mercury and other contaminants. Plus, they taste great—compared to tuna, I think salmon tastes richer and meatier, and therefore makes a better salad ingredient or dinner entrée.

Canned Alaska salmon is available at most supermarkets and wholesale clubs, such as Costco, and the pink, keta, and sockeye varieties of canned Alaska salmon can be very affordable. You can use it just like you'd use tuna. Some versions have skin and bones included, but they're soft, totally edible, and extranutritious. And there are widely available skinless and boneless versions, too.

Note: I usually steer clear of salmon that's not from Alaska or the Pacific Northwest. I avoid farmed salmon and Atlantic salmon, for example, because they tend to have a higher risk of contaminants and/or being harvested in eco-unfriendly ways. And believe it or not, that pink you see in farmed salmon is often from the addition of dyes!

Health Optimizer 6: Dial Down the Sodium, Pump up the Flavor

In my twenties, I had borderline high blood pressure, and I couldn't figure out why. So in my thirties, I dealt with the problem mostly by avoiding it. Then one day I had a break in my schedule at the ER and thought, "This is ridiculous. You're a doctor. Check your blood pressure already! How bad can it be?" After all, I was in good physical shape, worked out a lot, and thought my eating was superhealthy.

I wrapped a blood pressure monitor cuff around my arm, started pumping, and watched the digital numbers count down to the moment of truth. I was shocked. The numbers read 142 over 91. I thought, "This has to be a mistake!" I waited until later in the day when things were less hectic, tried to relax, and repeated the process. To my dismay, the numbers read 141 over 90. I realized I had a problem—anything over 140 over 90 is considered high blood pressure.

The problem, it turned out, was what I was eating. I was consuming way too much sodium in my everyday diet.

I was raised in a salt-loving culture. In my family, we shook salt onto everything. What's the first thing you do with a steak? Blast it with the salt shaker! See a baked potato? Throw salt on it. Salad? Give it a shot of salt. Scrambled eggs? Don't even think about it—give 'em some salt. It's the American way, and I was a true salt lover from the heartland.

While my affection for the salt shaker was bad enough, you know what the biggest culprit for me was? Frozen dinners and frozen pizzas. I ate them like they were going out of style. I thought they were healthy because I ate the kind that were loaded with veggies and lower in fat, but it turned out they were bursting with too much sodium.

The basic rundown on sodium intake is very simple, and according to health authorities like the American Heart Association and the Institute of Medicine, here are the basics:

- Your body needs sodium to function properly. Sodium is present in some amount naturally in most foods in their unprocessed state.

- But when you eat too much sodium, you raise your risk for high blood pressure, which in turn raises the risk for heart attack and stroke. (See page 126 for more information on blood pressure.)

- Adults should consume less than 2,300 milligrams of sodium per day, which is the equivalent of only a teaspoon.

- People over fifty, African Americans, and people with high blood pressure should consume less than 1,500 milligrams of sodium per day.

Americans consume over 3,400 milligrams of sodium per day on average, which has helped create a national health epidemic of high blood pressure. If we cut our sodium intake in half, says the National Heart, Lung, and Blood Institute, about 150,000 American lives could be saved every year.

The problem is not just the salt shaker, which only accounts for about 10 percent of the sodium we consume. The other 90 percent comes from sodium that's added to the packaged and processed foods we get at the supermarket—and the takeout and restaurant food we eat. Restaurant and food companies are dumping wildly excessive amounts of sodium into much of our food, making it very easy for us to go way over our daily recommended amount without even knowing it.

Although food manufacturers are starting to cut back on the amount of sodium they add to the nation's food supply, there are many supermarket items that still feature way too much of it. Here's just a sampling of the sodium hidden in some prepackaged meals (brand names have been withheld and lower sodium versions may be available):

Sample Supermarket Sodium Shockers	
Product	Sodium per serving (milligrams)
Buffalo Style Chicken Strips frozen dinner	2,060
Supreme Pizza for One (frozen)	1,450
Chicken Parmigiana & Penne frozen skillet meal	1,330
Beef Stew with Fresh Potatoes and Carrots (microwavable bowl)	1,250
Frozen Pepperoni Pizza for One	1,190
Beef with Country Vegetables (canned soup)	1,150
Meat Loaf and Gravy with Creamy Mashed Potatoes and Vegetables Frozen Dinner	1,120
Salisbury Steak Frozen Dinner	1,090
Roasted Chicken Flavored Rice with Carrots and Herbs (microwavable pouch)	1,020

The problem can be even worse with restaurants and takeout food. Although I primarily eat at home, I happen to like eating in restaurants, but I carefully watch what I eat when I go out. When I'm not taping *The Doctors* in Los Angeles, I live and work in Nashville, Tennessee, which has become a very eclectic town. If you're near Vanderbilt Medical Center where I work, you can walk in any direction and find really healthy food options. But out toward Opryland, it is a nutritional wasteland, as it is in so many parts of our country—mostly fast-food outlets and gas station mini-marts selling awful processed-foodlike substances and supersized megameals drenched in excess sodium and saturated fat.

It can be almost impossible to eat healthy in America when the restaurant choices all around us are so unhealthy. For many people, the majority of their caloric intake comes from restaurants, fast food, and takeout food. And usually that food is packed with ridiculously high levels of heart-unhealthy saturated fat and sodium.

A lifetime of eating too much sodium, which is the way many Americans are living, can inflict serious damage to a body. And in an elderly person, consuming a very high amount of sodium in just a single meal can raise the risk of congestive heart failure.

Here are just a few examples of the most egregiously high-sodium choices available at some of the top restaurant chains in America as of the time of the writing of this book. This is by no means a complete list, and some restaurants may offer lower-sodium versions of these dishes, but here is just a small sampling of some of the worst choices from a health standpoint at certain popular chain restaurants (the names of the restaurants have been omitted).

Restaurant Sodium Shockers

Product	Sodium per serving (milligrams)
Seafood Platter with Caesar Salad, Creamy Lobster-Topped Mashed Potato, Cheddar Biscuit, and a glass of lemonade	7,106
Buffalo Chicken Fajitas with tortillas, condiments, and a soda	6,916
Lasagna with a Breadstick, Garden Fresh Salad with House Dressing, and a soda	6,176
Quesadilla Burger	4,410
Buffalo Chicken Sandwich	2,300
Deluxe Breakfast (regular size biscuit) without syrup or margarine	2,150
Chicken Sandwich on French Bread	2,570
Chicken Cobb Salad Sandwich	1,340

Biggest Shocker: Children's meal combinations at America's largest chain and fast-food restaurants. The vast majority of these meals are too high in calories (93 percent over a reasonable target of 430 calories) too high in sodium (86 percent), and 45 percent of which are too high in saturated fat, according to a 2008 study by Center for Science in the Public Interest. Why is this alarming? Because a quarter of kids between five and ten are showing early signs of heart disease like elevated LDL (also known as "bad" cholesterol), or higher blood pressure.

The restaurant companies, under pressure from health officials, Congress, and advocacy groups like Center for Science in the Public Interest, are starting to make nutritional information more widely available, which is great news. It's not their job to make healthy choices for us, but they've got to do a better job of serving us food that is both delicious and healthier—and we've got to demand that they do, by insisting on reading key nutritional information like calories, sodium, and saturated fat before we order, and by voting with our pocketbooks and making better choices.

That day in the ER with the blood pressure monitor was a huge, fairly frightening wake-up call for me.

I was only thirty-four years old, thought I was a model of good health, and yet without even knowing it I was developing a high-risk factor for heart disease and stroke. Sodium was one thing I'd never paid any attention to, and from that point forward, I resolved to keep an eye on how much sodium I consumed, and I started by paying attention to the sodium counts on the nutrition labels of all the packaged food I ate.

You won't find a salt shaker in my house anymore. You won't find many processed foods either, which often contain too much sodium. I've learned to love firing up my food with garlic, herbs, pepper, and mustard—all kinds of healthy, delicious alternatives to salt. And you know what? I think my food tastes better now! The taste of garlic has become exponentially more appealing to me than the taste of salt. I still occasionally enjoy the healthier versions of frozen pizzas and frozen dinners, but now I always check the sodium count before I buy. And not surprisingly, my blood pressure has gone completely back to normal. I was 118 over 78 the last time I checked.

My numbers dropped twenty points from a simple diet change. I don't overstress about it either. When I occasionally eat high-sodium foods or meals, I'll keep an extra eye on my sodium intake the rest of the day and the next few days, so it all balances out. I adopted a simple, positive lifestyle habit and enjoyed a huge health benefit, and I know you can do the same! And don't think you can't reprogram your taste buds to enjoy less salt. It can take a little time and a little experimentation with alternatives, but your palate will come around and the health payoff is terrific. Take it from someone who ate too much salt for many years—you can totally do it!

Quick and Easy Tips for Lowering Your Sodium Intake

- Check food packages in the supermarket, ask for nutritional information at restaurants, and keep in mind one simple number: less than 2,300 milligrams of sodium per day, or less than 1,500 milligrams a day if you are over fifty, are African American, or have high blood pressure.
- Give the salt shaker a rest. Instead, spice up your food with pepper, mustard, garlic, lemon, herbs, and spices. Many supermarkets now have sections devoted to salt alternatives—check them out and experiment. I bet you'll easily find some options you'll love.

Health Optimizer 7: Upgrade Your Fats

For years, the idea of a low-fat diet was assumed to be a healthy one. The food industry sold us billions of dollars of low-fat products, but we kept getting fatter as we neglected the importance of how many total calories we took in. One day a study came out suggesting that the high-saturated-fat Atkins diet performed a little better than others for weight loss after a year. Then the Atkins approach was accused of increasing our risk for heart disease.

While delving into the best research on the subject, I was startled by how little we know for sure. As with most nutrition research, very little is based on the gold standard of randomized clinical trials. We are instead left with a lot of educated observations and speculations.

The good news, however, is that scientists are piecing together thousands of bits of evidence that point to one firm conclusion: for optimal health, you've got to have some fat on your plate! Dietary fats provide you with energy, help you absorb vitamins A, D, E, and

K, and help regulate a wide range of your body's functions. And let's face it, a little bit of fat makes meals tastier.

The evidence strongly suggests that to Eat to Savor Life and maximize your health, you should not focus on a high-fat or low-fat eating pattern, both of which I consider useless oversimplifications, but instead on getting high-quality fats on your plate in the right balance.

As long as you keep your total fat consumption at 20 to 35 percent of your calorie intake (personally, I shoot for under 30 percent), and you focus on the right kinds of fat, you're on the right track. As is the case with many things in life, you want the high-quality stuff. Just as your body needs "good" carbs from foods like whole grains, your body needs "good" fats. Good fats help protect you against a heart attack and bad fats can elevate the risk. Here's a rundown on what to avoid and what to enjoy:

──────────

Bad fats are saturated fat and trans fat. Saturated fat comes largely from animal sources like beef, poultry, and dairy. Trans fat comes largely from processed foods, including partially hydrogenated vegetable oils, margarine, French fries, and commercially baked crackers, cookies, cakes, and pies—though fortunately trans fat is being steadily reduced in the U.S. food supply.

Both saturated fats and trans fats can raise your risk of getting heart disease, by elevating both your total cholesterol and LDL ("bad") cholesterol (see page 127 for more on good and bad cholesterol). Trans fat has the double-whammy of also lowering HDL ("good") cholesterol. A steady diet of trans fat is absolutely terrible from a health standpoint. It's so bad for you that even though I usually preach everything in moderation, I absolutely refuse to eat anything that I know contains trans fat.

A third potentially bad fat, known as dietary cholesterol, is technically not a fat, but it's often grouped with the bad fats since it also elevates the artery-clogging cholesterol in your blood, though not as much as saturated fat or trans fat.

––––––––––

Good fats, by contrast, are monounsaturated fat and polyunsaturated fat, which includes omega-3 fatty acids. Good fats are believed to protect against heart disease and may offer other health benefits. Most of your dietary fat should come from sources of polyunsaturated and monounsaturated fatty acids, such as fish, nuts, and vegetable oils.

But if you're like me and you don't have time to whip out a calculator and figure out the fat percentages when you shop and eat out, you can in general follow the rule of thumb that I do: cover two-thirds or more of your plate with vegetables, fruit, whole grains, and beans, and one third or less with a lean protein source that's low in saturated fat.

That doesn't mean every meal you eat has to add up this way, it's just a very good overall pattern to aim for.

Simple Tips for Upgrading Your Fats

- Enjoy sources of good fats:

  - Extra virgin olive oil*

  - Canola oil

  - Avocados

––––––––––

* The FDA has approved a health claim for olive oil that consuming around 2 tablespoons daily may reduce the risk of heart disease. Extra-virgin olive oil is considered by many to be the most beneficial kind.

- ■ Walnuts

- ■ Fatty fish like salmon, sardines, mackerel, trout, and farmed oysters

- ■ High oleic safflower and sunflower oils

- ■ Flaxseeds and flax oil

- If you buy meat, dairy, or poultry products, minimize saturated fat by checking nutritional information and make choices that are lean, low fat, or fat free.

- Check nutritional information at the supermarket and restaurant, and choose items with zero trans fats.

- Remember that all sources of fat contain calories, so avoid consuming overly large amounts.

Health Optimizer 8: Switch Out Added Sugars

I used to drink soda all the time. I'd pop a soda with a sandwich during lunch, chug one with dinner, and guzzle another while watching TV.

Sweetened soft drinks were a perfectly normal part of my lifestyle, and over the years my palate became trained to accept a huge amount of sugar as a normal feeling. But as I got a little older, I also got frustrated with the money I was wasting on soda. I read the research on the negative health effects of excessive added sugars. And I gradually switched to good old-fashioned water.

And by old-fashioned water, I mean the kind that comes out of a tap. I consider the majority of sugar-spiked, vitamin-enhanced products and sports drinks to be an unnecessary use of money for most people. If you're an endurance athlete or you exercise regularly, you certainly may benefit from the replenished sodium, sugar, and electrolytes offered by a sports drink or vitamin-enhanced water. But most of us are drinking these beverages while sitting at our desks and the only thing they are doing is adding to our collective waistlines.

Today, I hardly ever drink soda or beverages with added sugars, except on rare occasions. In fact, I can barely drink them anymore, as they taste oversweet! You'll hardly ever find them in my refrigerator, and there's no reason you should waste your money on these empty calories either.

ASK DR. STORK

Question: Are energy drinks with caffeine really that bad for me?

Answer: In excess, yes, they are absolutely bad for you. There are lots of reasons why: drinks that contain too many calories from sugar can lead to weight problems; too much caffeine can lead to insomnia, and even in some cases, high blood pressure and anxiety; some of these "energy drinks" may even contain other stimulants or ingredients whose effects are not well understood yet.

If that doesn't deter you, consider this: I once had a trucker come into the ER after downing a number of these drinks during an overnight drive. He had a rapid heart rate and was drenched in sweat—he thought he was having a heart attack!

Remember, caffeine and other stimulants in these drinks are essentially drugs, and too much is bad for you. Keep your caffeine intake below 300 milligrams a day (or the equivalent of two or three small cups of coffee), and limit your intake in the afternoon and evening.

The Bottom Line: Minimize your consumption of so-called energy drinks containing caffeine and other stimulants. If you want a great energizing drink, go for water.

Sugar is a good thing. It tastes great, your body needs it, and moderate amounts of naturally occurring sugar in things like fruit, milk, and yogurt are absolutely okay. But America has gone completely overboard with consuming vast amounts of added sugars. Sweetened soda has become an American staple in many homes. It's considered absolutely normal to stock the fridge with gigantic bottles of sugar-spiked, artificially flavored and colored, green, orange, red, and caramel-colored water.

Stop and think about this: a typical 12-ounce can of orange soda contains 11 teaspoons of added sugar! The popular 20-ounce bottles that are frequently found in grab-and-go beverage cases in stores and soda machines boast 250 calories and almost 17 teaspoons of added sugar. How did that become a normal way of life? Would you ever dream of sitting down at the table with a spoon and a pile of sugar and eating 17 teaspoons of sugar, or feeding that much sugar to your child? That's what we're doing when we drink this stuff.

Sugar is added to lots of food products, like candy, cakes, cookies, pies, and chocolate milk. But the biggest category of food with added sugars in America is beverages, which are responsible for about 45 percent of total added sugars. This includes soft drinks and fruit drinks like fruit punch. And it has created a major health problem. According to researchers at the Harvard School of Public Health:

- "Strong evidence shows that sugary drinks are an important contributor to the epidemic rise of obesity and type 2 diabetes in the United States."

- Four out of five children and two out of three adults drink sugar-sweetened beverages on a typical day.

- A study of the health of 90,000 women over twenty years found that "women who drank more than two servings of sugary beverages each day had a nearly 40 percent higher risk of heart disease than women who rarely drank sugary beverages."

- Even diet drinks may not be a good replacement for sugary beverages. The research is mixed. While some studies suggest diet drinks promote weight control, there is also troubling evidence that regular use of artificial sweeteners could instead encourage weight gain. One reason: "For some, the consumption of calorie-reduced beverages could serve as justification for consumption of excess calories from other food sources."

- By choosing healthier beverages, you can decrease the risks to your health. (This is good news!)

I consider sugary beverages to be enormous wastes of money. These truly are empty calories that have a negative impact on both your wallet and your health. It's a real problem for children and adolescents, since soft drinks, containing almost zero nutrition, probably displace a nutritious alternative like milk, which boasts protein, vitamins and minerals like calcium, vitamin D, and vitamin A.

Sugar-sweetened beverages provide little or no nutritional benefit, they don't help us feel full like more nutritious beverages and foods, and they may displace those more nutritious choices from our diet. High-fructose corn syrup (HFCS), a sugar-containing sweetener used in many soft drinks, has been accused of presenting a higher risk of weight gain and diabetes than other sweeteners, but the research case for that has not been conclusively proven. The big problem in our eating patterns is way too much added sugars of all kinds, including HFCS.

Quick Tips for Reducing the Amount of Added Sugar in Your Diet

- Gradually replace sugary drinks with beverages like water, tea, herbal tea, and low-fat milk.

- Realize that water is great as an all-purpose everyday drink. It's free. It should be your go-to beverage.

- Instead of stocking your fridge with sugary drinks, add a few shots of 100 percent fruit juice, cucumbers, or lemon and lime twists to a quart of water and chill it overnight. Enjoy your naturally flavored water all day long.

- Look for foods and beverages with less added sugars on the ingredient list. Note that added sugars go by these different names: sugar, invert sugar, corn sweetener, corn syrup, high-fructose corn syrup, maltose, dextrose, malt syrup, fructose, molasses, fruit juice concentrates, glucose, sucrose, cane juice, and maltodextrin.

ASK DR. STORK

Question: How much water should I drink every day?

Answer: There's no one-size-fits-all answer to this question. It can depend on your physical activity, your sex, how hot your climate is, your diet, and your specific health conditions.

You, in large part, are made of water. Water is your number one chemical ingredient, accounting for about 60 percent of your body weight. Water provides your body a solvent for biochemical reactions, maintains vascular volume, helps supply nutrients to your tissues, and allows a conduit to clear out waste through the cardiovascular and digestive system. Even mild dehydration can sap your energy.

Water comes into your body not only from the fluids you drink, but the food you eat, which contributes roughly 20 percent of your water consumption. Lots of fruit and veggies, for example, can be up to 80 or 90 percent water by weight.

The idea of drinking "8 x 8," or at least eight 8-ounce glasses of water a day, has become a near-universal health commandment and almost a national habit. You see it in the media, on the internet, and in the advice from health authorities: "Drink at least eight glasses of water a day," with the recommendation usually aimed at healthy adults in a temperate climate leading a largely sedentary existence.

Between the late 1970s and the mid 1990s, consumption of all fluids per person in the U.S. jumped by roughly 20 percent, driven largely by a 25 percent increase in plain water, a doubling of soft drinks and alcohol, and an almost 2.5-fold increase in juices.

Then, in 2002, a funny thing happened.

The scientific *Journal of American Physiology* asked Heinz Valtin, MD, of the Dartmouth Medical School to search for the origins of the 8 x 8 recommendation. Ever since then, he's been looking for a well-designed scientific study that backs up the specific idea of 8 x 8. So far, he hasn't found a single one. Dr. Valtin can't even figure out for sure where the idea came from.

Although he found no scientific basis for 8 x 8 as advice for the entire population, Dr. Valtin did find evidence that large intakes of fluid, equal to and greater than 8 x 8, are advisable for the treatment or prevention of some diseases such as nephrogenic diabetes insipidus and renal stones, and "certainly are called for under special circumstances, such as vigorous work and exercise, especially in hot climates." He also found some evidence that a high water intake might reduce the risks for certain malignancies and of fatal coronary heart disease, but that further studies are needed to confirm the effects.

In rare circumstances, it's possible to drink too much water. For example, if a marathon runner or endurance athlete drinks very large amounts of water quickly and experiences an under-replacement of sodium, he or she is at higher risk of water intoxication and a life-threatening condition called hyponatremia. But this is typically associated with prolonged, stressful exercise lasting more than six hours, something relatively few people do. In even rarer circumstances, this can occur as a result of water-chugging contests.

The Bottom Line: As general rules of thumb, the Institute of Medicine recommends for adult women an average daily water intake of about 2.2 liters (about 9 cups), including drinking water. For adult men, the Institute recommends an average daily water intake of about 3.0 liters (about 13 cups), including drinking water. Pregnant women and breast-feeding women need additional fluids; the IOM recommends that pregnant women get 2.3 liters (about 10 cups) of water daily and women who breast-feed consume 3.1 liters (about 13 cups) per day.

You need more fluids if you engage in physical activity that makes you sweat, or you are in a hot climate. Experts at the Mayo Clinic estimate that an extra 1.5 to 2.5 cups of water should suffice for short bouts of exercise, but intense exercise for more than an hour requires more fluids.

Consult with your doctor or dietitian to estimate your specific water needs. (Bear in mind that some illnesses can require you consume more or less water than normal. Your doctor can advise you how to adjust your water intake if you are suffering from such an ailment.) Incidentally, the Institute of Medicine reports that while alcohol and caffeine-containing beverages have been shown in some studies to have diuretic effects, they may be transient in nature, and that such beverages in moderation should count as contributing to total water intake.

While there are guidelines, don't get too bogged down in these numbers. Unless you have an underlying medical problem that requires you to restrict your water intake, enjoy plenty of water throughout the day and you'll never have to worry about being dehydrated. To use a car analogy, keep your tank full so that when you do decide to go for that afternoon walk or run, you are well hydrated and won't sputter halfway through. Another rule of thumb: if your urine is always concentrated and dark, you may be underhydrating.

DR. STORK'S KEEP-IT-SIMPLE GUIDE TO READING NUTRITION INFORMATION (OR HOW TO MAKE BETTER CHOICES FOR OPTIMAL WELLNESS)

Let's face it; nutritional stats are a little complicated. Luckily, you don't have to take a calculator along with you when you shop or dine out to figure out what to buy or order. If you remember to keep your eye on a few key numbers, you can give your health a sharp boost. (And note that fruit and vegetables are so nutritious they hardly need nutrition labels! They're all good.)

Before I break down the stats to look out for on nutritional labels, here's a quick shortcut: If you follow the Eat to Savor Life mantra whenever you shop in the supermarket and fill your basket with many different kinds of whole veggies and fruit, whole grains, and healthy foods like fish, nuts, and beans, and minimize sodium, bad fats, added sugars and processed foods, the other nutrition label stats—vitamins, potassium, calcium, iron, cholesterol—will largely take care of themselves.

Top Stats to Pay Attention to on Food Packages and Restaurant Menus:

Calories: Most adults need only 2,000 to 2,800 calories a day. Very active people need more, and if you are trying to lose weight, you may need less. Calories matter a great deal for weight and health, so keep an eye on this number and try to shoot for your Personal Calorie Target each day (see page 135).

Sodium: To reduce the risk of high blood pressure, shoot for a daily total of under 2,300 milligrams per day, or under 1,500 milligrams a day if you are over fifty, or are African American or have high blood pressure.

Dietary Fiber: Shoot for a minimum 25 to 30 grams per day, from sources like beans, whole grains, and veggies.

Saturated Fat: Shoot for less than 20 grams total per day. The less of this, the better off you'll be. To keep your saturated fat intake down, reduce the amount of animal fats in your diet; if you consume dairy, make it low or no fat; eliminate fried foods from your diet; choose meats that are lean.

Total Fat: Shoot for less than 65 grams total per day. To help reduce blood cholesterol, your main source of fats should be from sources of good fat like fish, nuts, avocados, and corn, safflower, sunflower, olive, and canola oils.

Percentage of calories from fat: There is no universal number that experts agree on for what your percentage of calories from fat should be, but I shoot for less than 30 percent, with most of my fat calories coming from such foods as I mentioned above: nuts, healthy oils, and avocados. To figure out the percentage based on a nutritional label, take the calories from fat, then divide that number by total calories, and multiply the result by 100.

Trans fat: These are terrible for your health. Shoot for zero every day, or as close as possible to zero. To minimize your trans fat intake, cut out foods made with partially hydrogenated vegetable oils. The good news is that many American food manufacturers are pulling trans fats out of the food supply. Be aware that if a serving contains less than one half a gram of trans fat, the label will read zero. So avoid food items with "partially hydrogenated" in the ingredients list to ensure you eliminate deadly trans fats from your diet.

Cholesterol: Shoot for less than 300 milligrams per day. Some authorities suggest less than 200 milligrams.

Servings per container: Check this, as the numbers on the nutritional information label apply to one serving only. Lots of food packages contain more than one serving, so you may be eating more than you realize.

Ingredients: Look for products with short lists of ingredients. For bread and grain products, look for whole grain options by making sure the "whole" grain ingredient (whole wheat, whole rolled oats, brown rice, etc.) is the first on the list. Also, look for foods and beverages with little added sugars, which are listed as ingredients like brown sugar, invert sugar, corn sweetener, lactose, high fructose corn syrup, maltose, honey, dextrose, malt syrup, fructose, molasses, fruit juice concentrates, glucose, sucrose, cane juice, honey, and maltodextrin. Keep in mind the lower the ingredient is on the list, the less of it there will be in the product. Avoid partially hydrogenated oils.

The % Daily Values (DVs) on packaged food Nutrition Facts labels are considered general guidelines based on a 2,000-calorie daily intake. If your calorie needs are higher, then the percent listed on the label would be lower, and if your calorie needs are lower, then the percent listed will actually be higher. Calorie needs vary widely depending on someone's genetics, age, and activity level.

TRAVIS L. STORK, M.D.

℞   **EAT TO SAVOR LIFE:**
7 QUICK AND EASY TAKEAWAYS

1. Indulge in healthy eating patterns. Forget fad diets, deprivation, and guilt over food. Learn to fall in love with the healthy stuff, most of the time. Pamper yourself with nutrition knowledge—and occasional treats. Tweak your typical meal so that at least two-thirds of your plate is filled with vegetables, fruits, whole grains, and beans, and one-third or less is filled with a lean source of protein.

2. Enjoy many different kinds of whole veggies and fruit, all the time. The more fruits and vegetables in your life, the better. Load up your shopping cart with them and enjoy. Go for lots of variety and lots of colors.

3. Switch in the whole grains. Trade in your white refined grains for whole grains. Enjoy foods like oatmeal for breakfast, sandwiches on whole wheat and whole grain breads for lunch, and whole grain pasta and brown rice with dinner. Check the ingredient list to make sure that the whole grain is the first ingredient listed.

4. Enjoy more fish. Try omega-3-rich, eco-friendly options like Alaska salmon, Atlantic mackerel, sardines (U.S.), oysters (farmed), rainbow trout (farmed), arctic char (farmed), sablefish/ black cod (Alaska and Canada), and albacore tuna (U.S.). Use the fish lists on pages 62–63 to pick additional healthy choices.

5. Dial down the sodium, pump up the flavor. To reduce the risk of high blood pressure, shoot for a daily sodium total of under 2,300 milligrams per day, or under 1,500 milligrams a day if you are over fifty or are African American or have high blood

pressure. Give the salt shaker a rest. Instead, spice up your food with healthier options like pepper, mustard, garlic, lemon, herbs, and spices.

6. Upgrade your fats. Enjoy sources of good fats like extra virgin olive oil, canola oil, avocados, walnuts, and flaxseed. If you buy meat, dairy, or poultry products, minimize saturated fat by choosing lean, low fat, or fat free. Shoot for less than 20 grams total saturated fat per day. Look for choices with zero trans fats.

7. Switch out the added sugars. Cut back on the sodas and forget the sports drinks unless you're actually working out. Get a Bisphenol A-(BPA)-free water bottle and fill it up with cold water and enjoy it throughout the day. Lightly flavor your own water with a few slices of an orange, lemon, or lime if you want an extra kick.

DR. STORK'S INSTRUCTIONS

- Rip or copy this page out of the book and stick it on your refrigerator.
- Consult as often as needed.
- Discuss and review with your family, and your doctor.

THREE

GIVE YOUR BODY A DAILY VACATION

Close your eyes.

Try to imagine doing the most invigorating and mentally relaxing activity you can think of. Maybe it's waking up on a sunny summer morning and walking briskly on the beach or down a country lane. Maybe it's cross-country skiing with your whole family, shooting across a gorgeous winter landscape and sucking in the intoxicating, crisp winter air. Or it's autumn, and you're lightly jogging around a beautiful park in the city, your earphones streaming hypnotic, energetic tunes into your brain as leaves scatter in your wake. Perhaps you are kneeling in your garden in the springtime, your arms elbow deep in the soil as you yank up weeds and plant rows and rows of flowers, herbs, and vegetables. Or you might be dancing, swimming, biking, playing ball with your children, playing tennis, hiking, running, or shooting hoops.

In every one of these scenarios, you are doing two things that prove you have discovered one of the greatest secrets of a long, healthy, and happy life.

The first thing you're doing is you are sweating. That shows you've hopefully been moving for at least a half hour or so. Your heart is pumping faster than usual, your metabolism is revved up, endorphins are flowing through your bloodstream, your lungs are opening up, your brain is getting sharp and clear, and your muscles are enjoying a steady stream of extra warmth and oxygen.

The second thing is you are smiling.

Sure, you're enjoying the moment, but it's also something deeper. You are savoring physical activity that feels fantastic. You have found something you love to do. You are doing it not because you want to be as thin as you possibly can. You're not doing it out of a sense of grim determination or because you like to punish yourself. Quite the opposite. You're doing it because it feels so good. You would happily do it every chance you get, on most days of the week.

Technically, in these scenes you are doing what the vast majority of the world's best health experts say we all should be doing: thirty to sixty minutes of moderate to intense physical activity, most days of the week. But that's like saying a Picasso painting is "an aggregation of chemical-based pigments deposited on a stretched canvas platform."

What you're actually doing is giving your body and soul a Daily Physical Vacation.

That physical activity has got to be fun, or you won't want to do it most days of the week. And it's got to feel like a daily vacation, so you keep coming back for more.

In fact, every time you choose whether or not to be physically active, you are deciding how long and how well you want to live. If you don't get regular physical activity, you're going to increase your risk of heart disease, diabetes, and other diseases, including all the major killers. That's hard for people to grasp until they get to a point where it's too late. Unfortunately, over 55 percent of U.S. adults don't get any regular physical activity outside their normal routine.

But here's some wonderful news: giving your body an extremely fun daily physical vacation is one of the keys to optimal wellness. It's cheap, it's simple, and it can transform your entire life.

Now I'd like to write you one of the most important prescriptions you've ever received.

TRAVIS L. STORK, M.D.

℞

DR. STORK'S PRESCRIPTION FOR A
DAILY PHYSICAL VACATION (DPV)

To feel great, maintain a healthy weight, and optimize your health against a wide range of chronic diseases, pamper your body with a Daily Physical Vacation (DPV) of at least thirty to sixty minutes of moderate-intensity physical activity, most days of the week. Here's how:

- Try to break a sweat every day.
- Smile as often as possible while you're doing it.
- Don't have a "suffer-fest." Rather than punishing yourself, pamper yourself with physical activity that feels good.

Keep in mind:

- Your DPV should feel like the opposite of punishment—it should feel like a high-energy treat for your body. If one physical activity feels like a chore, skip it and try another. Remember, any time you start a new activity you're likely to be a little sore afterward, but it should get easier.
- Your DPV doesn't have to require a fitness club or expensive sports equipment: brisk walking for a half hour a day, or better yet an hour, counts as a near-perfect DPV: it delivers major health benefits, is ultracheap and supereasy.

This one simple lifestyle change can, over time, add years to your life, sharply boost the quality of your health, and make you feel wonderful physically and mentally.

Here are seven reasons for you to fall in love with regular physical activity and start planning DPVs:

Reason 1: A DPV is a free, multipurpose wonder drug with no side effects.

It effectively combats a wide range of illnesses. Unlike the vast majority of traditional medicines and alternative medicines, regular physical activity is virtually free and requires no medical insurance bureaucracy for reimbursement. It has almost no negative side effects, aside from the risk of an activity-related injury. Nobody, even if they believe the opposite, is allergic to physical activity!

Reason 2: DPV is the ultimate alternative medicine.

This claim is backed up by excellent research. Unlike the vast majority of so-called alternative medicines, it is proven to work. It is the ultimate expression of your independence and control, and your freedom from the medical establishment. You control the dosage, govern its effectiveness, and make it work through your enthusiasm and commitment.

Reason 3: DPV is nature's Lipitor.

According to the American Heart Association, an activity like walking for only thirty minutes on most days of the week can help reduce the risk of heart disease while improving blood cholesterol levels.

Reason 4: DPV is nature's Prozac.

A wide range of research indicates that regular physical activity can give you real psychological health benefits. Specifically, it can improve mood, relieve stress, protect against depression, reduce depressive symptoms, work as an effective complement to therapy and medication in cases of depression, and improve your feelings of self-esteem and well-being.

Reason 5: DPV is nature's Viagra.

Research suggests that regular physical activity in combination with other lifestyle factors such as healthy eating, smoking cessation, and a healthy weight may improve sexual function for both men and women.

Reason 6: DPV is a supervaccine against a wide range of chronic diseases.

The list of physical conditions that can be improved through regular physical activity, especially in combination with other lifestyle factors, is an extraordinary one. There is good evidence that it can:

- Lower risk for premature death

- Lower risk for heart attack and stroke

- Slow or reverse the progress of cardiovascular disease, and lower your risk of dying from it

- Improve blood lipid profile (a series of measurements of cardiovascular health)

- Lower risk for type 2 diabetes

- Lower risk for high blood pressure

- Improve overall quality of life

- Lower risk for colon and breast cancers, may reduce the risk of other cancers, and may deliver health benefits if you already have cancer

- Help maintain healthy weight, prevent weight gain, and, when combined with a healthy diet and calorie control, will help with weight loss and reduce abdominal obesity

- Improve cardiorespiratory and muscular fitness

- Help build and maintain bones, joints, muscle strength, and endurance; reduce risk for osteoporosis, falls, and hip fracture

- Reduce arthritis pain and associated disability

- Improve sleep quality

- Enhance flexibility and posture

- Improve body composition, improve autonomic nervous system function, reduce systematic inflammation, reduce blood coagulation, and improve coronary blood flow, vascular function, and cardiac function

- Encourage new brain cells, promote good blood flow to the brain, and protect against risk factors for Alzheimer's and other dementias.

Reason 7: DPVs are your biological destiny.

You are genetically programmed for daily physical activity. For tens of thousands of years, your ancestors were nomads and hunter-gatherers and eventually agrarian workers, constantly on the move, chasing, chopping, lifting, pushing, moving, and exerting themselves through their entire lives. It is biologically abnormal for you to be sitting on the couch watching TV for long periods of time.

Our genes evolved and adapted over ages of very high physical activity. Then, about a hundred years ago, the results of the industrial revolution suddenly removed the need for physical labor and activity from many people's lives. But guess what—our genes haven't changed. And too many of us spend much of our lives behind desks, in our cars, and sitting down with a remote control in our hands. The result is a major "disconnect" that damages our health and fuels chronic disease.

The good news is that a little physical activity goes a long way, particularly if you're just getting started. Generally speaking, the more physical activity you enjoy, the more health benefits you'll experience, but immediate temporary improvements in blood pressure and cholesterol occur with just one session, and even modest routines of physical activity deliver major health benefits to people who were previously sedentary. And for people who already have a chronic illness, regular physical activity may reduce its impact. For example, arthritis sufferers can enjoy more movement and less pain, type 2 diabetes patients can enjoy less heart disease risk, and patients with some types of cancer can enjoy increased longevity. While moderate-intensity physical activity delivers excellent health benefits, vigorous-intensity delivers even better results. But there's absolutely no reason you need to go to extremes. Overly severe and extreme physical activity can both trigger injuries and generate more oxidative stress and free radicals than the body can handle. A half hour or hour of moderate-intensity physical activity, most days of the week, is all anybody needs for optimal health. That approach, over time, is probably our healthiest option, and is sustainable over a lifetime.

You can choose to be an extreme athlete and climb Mount Everest, or become an Ironman triathlete, or swim the English Channel, run the Iditarod, or compete in an ultramarathon. Personally, I can't do an extremely intense two-hour workout after a long day working in the emergency room. For the average working person, it's unrealistic to expect that extremely intense exercise is a viable option. That's not to say you can't go out on some days and push yourself hard for two or three hours, but it's not necessary all the time for maximum health.

The key to fitness is to enjoy it.

I've never had a personal trainer in my life and I never will. I love making up my own workouts as I go along. However, for some people, hiring a personal trainer is a great way to get started exercising and help stay motivated. If you decide to work with a trainer, be sure to find someone who will make exercising a fun, positive experience for you. If you don't enjoy it and suffer through your exercise, you can become miserable, dejected, and depressed, and you'll give up. It's the same reason diets don't work. Constantly suffering through every workout is not sustainable, it's not necessary, and it's not the road to optimal wellness.

It's perfectly natural for your Daily Physical Vacation lifestyle to have peaks and valleys. There may be two or three days when you don't break a sweat. But that's no excuse for you not to go out and treat yourself the fourth day. Believe me; I've had days when I feel so exhausted from work, it's hard to even get off the couch to grab the phone to order dinner. I just have no energy to do anything but lie there! But a healthy mind-set has become so ingrained in my mind that I'll get out and get moving the next day.

My cohosts on *The Doctors* make fun of me for being a hard-core athlete, but I'm not really that hard-core. I don't believe in extreme exercise. I don't think it works for most people. I try to get to the gym at least three times a week for resistance work, otherwise known as strength training. I try to go for a longer bike ride a few times a week, and life is too short for me not to enjoy that bike ride. Biking is my hobby, and I love it. In addition to the health benefits I've outlined, biking is a huge stress reliever for me. Simply put, it makes me feel great. The goal of your Daily Physical Vacation isn't to be as thin as possible or to be as good-looking as possible, but to feel as fantastic as you possibly can.

My typical workout will depend on my mood, my energy levels, and how much time I have. I don't adhere to a rigid workout schedule, but I do shoot for an hour-long Daily Vacation on most days of the week. Some days it will turn into a three- or four-hour bike ride, and some days I'm not able to get any physical activity. I don't go to the gym and do overly rigorous training regimens that I can't sustain over time. I bicycle all the time, but I've never won a bike race, and I probably never will. For me, the victory is simply being on the bike for a few hours, or getting to the top of the mountain.

For some people, a rigid training schedule is all that works. For others, having a race on the upcoming schedule is the only thing that will motivate them to go running. And that's an important thing to remember: what works for me, or your spouse, or your best friend, may not work for you. So don't fret if you don't enjoy a certain activity the way your friends do. Just keep searching for an activity you do enjoy that provides you with your own daily vacation. If you are active and moving, that's all that matters!

The healthiest time in my life was when I lived in Colorado for several years as an adult. I found myself in a culture where it seemed everyone was physically active, and it really rubbed off on me. My friends and I didn't have a happy hour after work; instead, we'd go out for an intense mountain bike ride and then we'd enjoy a beer. And let me tell you, a cold beer never tasted better! I wound up mountain biking or white-water kayaking almost every day in the summer and cross-country skiing most days in winter.

Today, when I'm in Nashville, I try to ride my bike everywhere—to the hospital, to the grocery store, on errands. When I have time, I ride a twenty-five-mile loop out to a nearby park or take my dog on a hike. I'll still try to get to the gym for resistance training, but I'll preferentially choose outdoor activities like biking, jogging, or hiking. Conversely, when I'm working in Los Angeles taping *The Doctors,* I find it a lot harder to exercise outdoors due to my busy schedule, so I'm more dependent on the gym.

I own a stand-up paddleboard, and on hot summer days in Nashville I'll go jump in a lake and start paddling away. People look at me like I'm crazy, but I don't mind! I have a friend who lives right in the middle of Manhattan, so he stays in shape by jogging around Central Park every chance he gets. People in New York, it turns out, are pretty doggone lean and healthy, in large part because they're walking around so much. In Los Angeles, I recently discovered that the side streets are often empty, so that's where you'll find me on my bike. Whenever I'm back in Colorado in late spring, you'll find me in my white-water kayak, which is a fantastic, fun, and adrenaline-filled workout.

Simply put, I try to break a sweat every day, but just like you, I have to adjust my daily vacation to my location, my schedule, and the weather.

No matter where you live, you can find physical activities that you'll enjoy.

Physical activity does have one limitation: by itself, it's not very good at helping you lose weight. "In general, for weight loss, exercise is pretty useless," said exercise expert Eric Ravussin, chair in diabetes and metabolism at Louisiana State University, in a 2009 *Time* magazine cover story titled "Why Exercise Won't Make You Thin."

But physical activity is excellent for both overall health and for helping you keep weight off.

It is very hard to lose weight through physical activity alone. Exercise by itself doesn't seem to make much of a dent in our weight if we don't take into account what we eat. There is even a theory that exercise can make some people hungry to the point of overcompensating and overindulging in high-calorie foods. The lesson: don't reward yourself after a 300-calories-burned workout by wolfing down 500-plus calories' worth of a mocha and blueberry scone!

Weight loss occurs more effectively through improved eating habits. But increasing your physical activity is an excellent way to keep the pounds off. Physical activity, in other words, is the force multiplier of healthy eating. The Centers for Disease Control and Prevention explains it this way:

- "Most weight loss occurs because of decreased caloric intake. However, evidence shows the only way to maintain weight loss is to be engaged in regular physical activity."

- "When losing weight, more physical activity increases the number of calories your body uses for energy, or 'burns off.' The burning of calories through physical activity, combined with reducing the number of calories you eat, creates a 'calorie deficit' that results in weight loss."

But how much physical activity is needed to keep weight off? After all, many of us can lose weight, but then it creeps back up on us. In many cases, it turns out it's because we're just not moving enough: many experts agree that at least sixty to ninety minutes a day of moderate-intensity physical activity is needed to maintain a substantial weight loss.

One clue to the power of physical activity to help maintain weight loss lies with an extraordinary group of people who have figured out how to lose weight and keep it off. They are participants in a fascinating ongoing study called the National Weight Control Registry, or NWCR, created in 1993 by Rena Wing, PhD, of Brown Medical School, and James O. Hill, PhD, of the University of Colorado. It is a one-of-a-kind study of "successful losers": people who have lost at least thirty pounds for at least a year.

There are more than 5,000 people now being followed in the Registry, and on average they've kept about 70 pounds off for almost six years. How did they do it? Here are some of the most interesting findings:

Five Habits of Successful Losers

1. They get out and move—a lot: they engage in very high levels of physical activity: 94 percent of NWCR participants ramped up their physical activity, with the most popular activity being walking. 90 percent of them exercise, on average, about one hour per day.

2. They switch off the TV: 62 percent of Registry participants watch less than ten hours of TV per week.

3. They eat better: 98 percent report that they modified their food intake in some way to lose weight.

4. They don't skip breakfast: about 80 percent eat breakfast every day.

5. They keep an eye on the scale: 75 percent weigh themselves at least once a week.

BE YOUR OWN PERSONAL TRAINER (LET'S GET FIRED UP!)

Okay, it's pep-talk time.

One of the great things a personal trainer can do is to get you fired up and inspired to commit to physical activity. Some people need the structure, disciplines and enthusiasm a good personal trainer can offer. While I've seen people have tremendous results with personal trainers, having a personal trainer is absolutely not mandatory to succeed. You can fire yourself up just as powerfully and, with the proper knowledge and tools, you can be your own personal trainer.

The first big step is motivation. Now, there are lots of excuses for you to stay planted on the couch like a happy geranium. Believe me, I know them. I've been there on many a night myself.

A supercomfortable couch can be a bewitching, seductive place to be. A place where all the stresses in life melt away—the bills, the traffic, the dumb boss.

Well, I'm here to tell you to GET UP AND GO. You are not a Potato. You can enjoy the couch later, after you've broken a sweat.

The pleasant narcotic-like feeling you're having is a false, counterproductive, and medically dangerous pleasure—if you're not also enjoying regular physical activity in your life.

ASK DR. STORK

Question: Can I exercise if I'm sick?

Answer: It depends. How sick are you? My general rule of thumb is if all your symptoms are from the head up—primarily a runny/stuffy nose—then go ahead and enjoy a moderate workout, but not an intense one. If you have a basic head cold or congestion, moderate exercise shouldn't make your condition worse, and it can even make you feel better.

If your symptoms go below into your chest—for instance, if you have bronchitis and a major cough, or if you have flulike symptoms, fever, body aches, and chills—then rest, rest, rest!

You are not a root vegetable, destined to spend your years attached motionless to the soil as you stare at electronic impulses flickering on a screen.

You are a tiger. Your genes have predestined you to roam the open plains, explore the forests, climb hills, and swim streams. Your biological engineering is such that you are built to move, to jump, to climb, chase, and throw. You shouldn't try to escape or ignore this destiny—if you do, your body will fight back by increasing your risks of disease and premature death.

But if you embrace your destiny, get up, get moving, and break a sweat most days of the week, you will live longer, be healthier, and feel fantastic.

What's keeping you from doing this? I can think of some powerful excuses. You're working longer and harder. You have kids. You are taking care of your parents. Your bosses and clients have you on call on your BlackBerry or iPhone around the clock. The idea of trying to squeeze in extra time to exercise can sound like a cruel joke.

I hear these excuses all the time from my patients, and even from fellow doctors. But you must realize that you can find the time. More important, appreciate why you need to find time and what you're missing out on if you don't! Here are some tips for scheduling a Daily Physical Vacation:

Solution 1. Identify wasted time— and flip it into daily vacation time.

Let's stop for a moment and think about your day and about your week. What are you really spending time on?

I'll bet that if you try, you can identify an incredible amount of wasted time.

It could be the time you spent overchecking your email. It could be time you were vegetating on the couch watching TV. Or perhaps you slept in for a half hour for no particular reason. Or you wasted time unproductively on the internet, googling unimportant subjects and updating your "What's on your mind?" information.

The next time you get the urge to spend a half hour updating your Twitter account, your Facebook page, or cruising the web for no particular reason, just shut the computer off, get up, and take a light jog or a brisk power walk through the neighborhood.

By reprioritizing, almost anybody can find at least a half hour, most days of the week, to take a Daily Physical Vacation. Look at it this way: you don't have time to not take care of yourself!

Solution 2. Invite your spouse and/or family on a Daily Physical Vacation.

Think carefully about exactly how your whole family is spending its time. All those wasted minutes spent with electronic gizmos really adds up, right? When you eliminate all but the most essential computer and TV use (like watching *The Doctors*—ha!), I bet you, your spouse, and your kids will find at least a half hour to spare, many days of the week.

Next, inspire your family to commit to making physical activity a routine, automatic, no-big-deal part of your family schedule. On weekends, for example, lots of families either watch even more TV than usual, or they drive to the mall. Instead, take just thirty or sixty minutes of that time to take a power walk around the neighborhood with your spouse and kids, or toss a Frisbee around at the nearest park with your significant other.

If you can get your spouse or significant other to join you in physical activity, I think it will be a tremendous victory in your life. You will be much more likely to succeed. I've seen wonderful stories of spouses who both weighed in the 300-pound range, who committed to getting to a healthy weight together through healthy eating and physical activity, and they do it. These stories are amazing and inspiring to me, because the positive attitudes of these couples are so powerful. The shared experience and accomplishment is so empowering to them, and it does wonders for their relationships, too.

Create a mind-set in your family that physical activity is a built-in part of the daily routine.

Solution 3. Take all the shortcuts you can.

Naturally, it's easier to get moving if you have a gym, hiking trail, or park nearby, but those aren't always available. Lots of places in America barely have any sidewalks or anywhere to safely walk or bike. If that's the case in your town, what should you do?

Be creative, and take shortcuts. The key is to switch out little chunks of unproductive time and find windows of opportunity to squeeze in physical activity. You don't even have to leave the house to work out. Instead, try this ultracheap and easy approach:

The World's Simplest Killer Workout
(or, How to turn your TV room into an instant
micro-home-gym for everyday and rainy-day use)

- Get a good set of resistance bands (these cost as little as $30 at a sporting goods store or on the internet). They are handy, easy-to-use elastic sheets that can deliver the same strength training benefits as an elite gym.

- Do a resistance workout by rotating through the exercises indicated in the brochures that come with the bands.

- March vigorously in place or jump rope while you watch your favorite TV shows or DVDs. For marching in place, swing your arms and get your knees up high. Your pace and energy level should be equal to a brisk walk. Start with five minutes, then work yourself up to thirty minutes or more. You should break a sweat.

- Congratulations! You've pampered yourself with a nearly perfect entry-level workout that combines cardiovascular and strength training, and you're delivering excellent health benefits to your body and mind.

- Stick with it, and over time expand your repertoire.

Solution 4. Turn social dates into activity dates.

Is it just me, or do you think we make too many social dates that are centered on drinking alcohol and eating unhealthy food? Although I've been guilty of playing along, I never understood that! So many of our weekday lunches with friends or colleagues are based on sitting down indoors for an hour or two, stuffing ourselves with a huge lunch, and then feeling sleepy all afternoon. Many people seem to automatically plan their weekend with friends around gorging on things like killer margaritas and greasy food. I constantly overhear people describe an enjoyable weekend with the phrase "I got sooo drunk!" Sure, alcohol and junk food can feel good temporarily, and if you throw in some dancing I guess you're getting a workout of sorts, but why don't we get a little creative?

Instead, I love to make physical activity dates with my friends. You can even do it for business meetings—I once went on a rafting trip with my co-workers, and it was one of the most productive professional bonding experiences I have ever experienced.

At lunchtime, go for a thirty-minute brisk walk with your co-worker. Invite your friends out for a bike ride or a game of Frisbee. Just because you aren't a kid anymore shouldn't mean you no longer get to play! Take your significant other on a hike and bring along a healthy picnic. In all these cases, you'll probably make a deeper emotional connection with the people you're with, because you're adding the huge dimension of physical activity, and the energy, pleasure, and endorphins it delivers.

ASK DR. STORK

Question: I'm afraid of getting injured if I increase my level of physical activity. Also, someone told me if I exercise I could have a heart attack. Is increasing my physical activity level potentially dangerous?

Answer: Adults of all sizes and shapes gain health and fitness benefits by being habitually physically active, and for virtually everyone the many benefits of regular physical activity outweigh the risks of injury and sudden heart attacks.

In 2008, a major 643-page expert report was published that synthesized all the latest, best research on the health benefits of physical activity. Commissioned by the federal government, the document is called *Physical Activity Guidelines for Americans.*

According to this major research review conducted by scientific and medical experts, moderate-intensity physical activity like brisk walking has a low risk of adverse events. Here's how the experts break it down:

- The risk of musculoskeletal injury does increase with the total amount of physical activity. For example, a person who regularly runs 40 miles a week has a higher risk of injury than a person who runs 10 miles each week. However, people who are physically active may have fewer injuries from other causes, such as motor vehicle collisions or work-related injuries. Depending on the type and amount of activity that physically active people do, their overall injury rate may be lower than the overall injury rate for inactive people.
- Participation in contact or collision sports, such as soccer or football, obviously involves a higher risk of injury than participation in noncontact physical activity, such as swimming or walking. However, when performing the same activity, people who are less fit are more likely to be injured than people who are fitter.
- Cardiac events, such as a heart attack or sudden death during physical activity, are rare. However, the risk of such cardiac events does increase when a person suddenly becomes much more active than usual. The greatest risk occurs when an adult who is usually inactive engages in a vigorous-intensity activity

like shoveling snow. People who are regularly physically active have the lowest risk of cardiac events both while being active and overall.

- Very high levels of physical activity may have extra risks, but we are talking about athletes who engage in what many would call extreme levels of activity.

The Bottom Line: The health benefits of physical activity far outweigh the risks of adverse events for almost everyone.

3 SIMPLE PHRASES—AND 1 MAGIC FORMULA

The world of fitness and exercise can seem really complicated. If you're not a hard-core fitness buff, you can get bewildered by the multitude of technical terms that are thrown around in gyms and health clubs. Circuit training, interval training, creatine, glucosamine, target heart rates, anaerobic thresholds . . . what does it all mean?

The good news is that for everyday optimal wellness, you can skip the jargon and focus mainly on three simple phrases and one magic formula. They are all you really need to know.

The three magic phrases are moderate aerobic activities, vigorous aerobic activities, and resistance exercises.

———

Moderate aerobic activities are performed at an intensity that gets your heart beating faster than normal, usually causing you to break a sweat. You can still carry on a conversation, but you would find it hard to sing a song. A classic example is brisk walking. Talking on your cell phone while walking slowly on a treadmill that's set to two miles an hour doesn't count! I've got friends who say they exercise, but when I see them in action, they're not even breaking a sweat. It's better than nothing, but they wonder why they're not feeling the health benefits. The reason? They're not moving fast enough.

Examples of moderate-intensity aerobic activities include:

- Brisk walking—3 or 4 miles an hour

- Biking around 10 miles per hour

- Ballroom and line dancing

- Canoeing (you have to actually paddle!)

- Gardening and yardwork—raking, trimming shrubs

- Catch-and-throw sports—baseball, softball, volleyball

- Active play with your children (Frisbee, spongeball sports)

- Golf, including walking and carrying clubs

- Using hand cyclers (also called ergometers)

- Water aerobics

Vigorous aerobic activities make your breathing rapid and raise your heart rate substantially. You can speak only a couple of words without losing your breath. Examples of vigorous intensity activities include:

- Aerobics

- Biking—10 miles per hour or faster

- Fast dancing

- Heavy gardening (continuous digging or hoeing)

- Martial arts like karate

- Race walking, running, or jogging—at least 5 miles an hour

- Sports with a lot of running (basketball, football, soccer)

- Swimming laps

- Tennis (singles)

- Rollerblading/in-line skating briskly

- Jumping rope

Resistance exercises are also called **muscle-strengthening exercises** and **strength-building activities.**

I think it's a shame that more people, especially women, don't engage in resistance exercises. Many people don't understand how crucial these exercises are to our health. "Lifting weights" seems to connote an optional, vanity-type activity, but resistance training helps your body achieve optimal function and prevents injuries and fractures as we get older.

Resistance exercises provide an excellent way to help us keep weight off over the long haul. They are great for preventing bone loss, and are a real help to getting to an optimal body weight. The reason: more muscle = higher metabolism = you're burning more calories, even while you sleep. Examples include:

- Calisthenics like push-ups and pull-ups

- Exercise bands (elastic strips)

- Weight machines

- Handheld free weights

- Any activity that is building muscle, such as rock climbing

Note: Remember to warm up and cool down. Experts at the University of California-Berkeley suggest: "Slowly jog for five minutes before your workout to gradually increase your heart rate and core temperature. Cool down after exercising with five minutes of slower-paced movement. This prevents an abrupt drop in blood pressure and helps alleviate potential muscle stiffness." Experts agree it's a bad idea to do static stretching before exercising, so always warm up before stretching, or save stretching until after you exercise.

The report *Physical Activity Guidelines for Americans* concludes that both aerobic activities and resistance activities are essential to our health—combining aerobic activity with resistance activity is your best bet for long-term optimal weight levels and optimal health. The experts identified the two major levels of physical activity that deliver health benefits, or what I call "thresholds":

The Major Health Benefits Threshold. Substantial health benefits are achieved when adults sixteen to sixty-four reach a total amount of 150 minutes, or 2 hours and 30 minutes, of moderate-intensity aerobic activity per week.

As an option, the same benefits are achieved by reaching a total amount of 75 minutes, or 1 hour and 15 minutes, of vigorous intensity aerobic activity per week—or by the equivalent combination of moderate and vigorous aerobic activities.

Most health benefits occur at this threshold point of physical activity, according to the research. But extra benefits do kick in at a higher level.

The Extra Benefits Threshold. Additional and more extensive health benefits are achieved when an adult reaches a total amount of 300 minutes (5 hours) a week of moderate-intensity aerobic activity, or 150 minutes a week of vigorous-intensity aerobic activity; or the equivalent combination of the two. Even more benefits are gained by engaging in physical activity beyond these amounts. You get the idea: more is better but a little goes a long way!

I've boiled all the best research and recommendations down for you, including the federal guidelines and the latest advice of the American College of Sports Medicine and the American Heart Association, and created the following plan for you to get the most health benefits from physical activity.

DR. STORK'S MAGIC FORMULA: PHYSICAL ACTIVITY VACATIONS FOR OPTIMAL WELLNESS

Simple version: For major health benefits, get at least 30 to 60 minutes of moderate-intensity aerobic activity, like brisk walking, on most days of the week. (Note that at least 60 to 90 minutes of moderate-intensity aerobic activity on most days of the week may be needed to prevent regaining weight for the formerly overweight or obese.)

Detailed version: Do a minimum of 2 hours and 30 minutes of moderate-intensity aerobic activity a week—*or* 1 hour and 15 minutes (75 minutes) a week of vigorous-intensity aerobic physical activity, *or* an equivalent combination of the two. Activity should be performed in episodes of at least 10 minutes, preferably spread throughout the week.

Also, on at least 2 days a week, do resistance activities that involve all the major muscle groups. A goal, for example, might be 8 to 12 repetitions of 6 to 8 strength-training exercises. One set is effective, but some evidence suggests that 2 or 3 sets may be more effective.

A WEEK OF SAMPLE PHYSICAL VACATIONS FOR MAJOR HEALTH BENEFITS

The following examples, based on the *2008 Physical Activity Guidelines for Americans,* show how it's possible to hit the major health benefits threshold by getting the equivalent of 150 minutes (2 hours and 30 minutes) of moderate-intensity aerobic physical activity a week, plus resistance activities. I think you'll agree that these plans sound like fun!

- 30 minutes of brisk walking (moderate intensity) on 5 days, exercising with resistance bands (resistance) on 2 days
- 25 minutes of running (vigorous intensity) on 3 days, lifting weights (resistance) on 2 days

---

- 30 minutes of brisk walking on 2 days, 60 minutes (1 hour) of social dancing (moderate intensity) on 1 evening, 30 minutes of mowing the lawn (moderate intensity) on 1 afternoon, heavy gardening (resistance) on 2 days
- 30 minutes of an aerobic dance class on 1 morning (vigorous intensity), 30 minutes of running on 1 day (vigorous intensity), 30 minutes of brisk walking on 1 day (moderate intensity), calisthenics (such as sit-ups, push-ups) on 3 days (resistance)
- 30 minutes of biking to and from work on 3 days (moderate intensity), playing softball for 60 minutes on 1 day (moderate intensity), using weight machines on 2 days (resistance)
- 45 minutes of doubles tennis on 2 days (moderate intensity), lifting weights after work on 1 day (resistance); hiking vigorously for 30 minutes, and rock climbing (resistance) on 1 day

ASK DR. STORK

Question: I've got a medical condition. It is safe for me to exercise?

Answer: I hear things like this all the time from patients: "I have arthritis/heart disease/bad knees, so I can't exercise."

In many cases, the opposite is true. They should exercise.

Many people think that if you've got a medical condition, you really ought to lay off the exercise. But, in fact, regular physical activity and structured exercise, under a doctor's supervision, is usually a great idea.

For cancer survivors, for example, physical activity may help increase quality of life, reduce adverse effects of cancer treatments, and reduce the risk of developing other conditions, as cancer survivors are living longer and longer these days. Also, studies suggest that physically active adults with colon or breast cancer have a reduced risk of the cancer recurring, or of premature death. People with type 2 diabetes are routinely prescribed physical activity by their doctors—sometimes, along with dietary changes, that is the only treatment needed. Heart disease patients are often counseled with the same prescription—the benefits almost always outweigh the risks.

Many people who suffer from the fatigue and pain of osteoarthritis worry that physical activity could make things worse. But according to the government's *2008 Physical Activity Guidelines for Americans,* "Strong scientific evidence indicates that both aerobic activity and muscle-strengthening activity provide therapeutic benefits for persons with osteoarthritis. When done safely, physical activity does not make the disease or the pain worse." The likely payoff: less pain, better physical function and mood, and quality of life. Health-care providers typically counsel people with osteoarthritis to do lower impact activities like swimming, walking, and strength training.

Adults with disabilities can also benefit from regular physical activity, including stroke victims, people with spinal cord injury, multiple sclerosis, Parkinson's disease, muscular dystrophy, cerebral palsy, traumatic brain injury, limb amputations, mental illness, and dementia. The payoffs include improved cardiovascular fitness and better mental health.

Healthy pregnant women benefit from moderate-intensity physical activity, too, with an overall health and cardiorespiratory fitness boost. The benefits to the woman continue after a normal birth, by enhancing baseline fitness, helping maintain a healthy weight, and elevating her mood. Risks from such activity are low. Pregnant women should not do exercises involving lying on their backs after the first trimester, and should also avoid doing activities that could increase the risk of falling or abdominal trauma, such as contact or collision sports like horseback riding, skiing, soccer, and basketball. Think low-impact activities if you're pregnant. Certainly discuss any concerning activity with your ob-gyn.

The Bottom Line: I don't care what your physical condition is—you and your doctor should be able to find a moderate- to vigorous-intensity physical activity that you will love to do regularly that is both safe and effective.

Give Your Body a Daily Vacation: 10 Quick and Easy Takeaways

Hopefully you're now sufficiently fired up and ready to embark on your life of DPVs. Please refer back to the tips below as you create and enjoy your own fitness plans:

- Consult your doctor before starting an exercise program.

- Realize that regular physical activity is your Miracle Drug for optimal wellness, providing a host of physical and mental benefits. It is your supervaccine against chronic disease.

- Remember it's never too late to get in shape. You can absolutely do it. And you absolutely will! Take charge, and get moving. I know you can do it!

- Know that your body is genetically programmed for daily physical activity—thousands of years of evolution is telling you to get out, get moving, and enjoy yourself.

- Make fitness your hobby, not a chore. It can become a passion that will enhance every aspect of your life, and something you'll never dream of giving up.

- Try to break a sweat every day, doing something you love. Know that you don't have to be an ultramarathoner to get the benefits of exercise.

- Start slowly and increase your time and intensity gradually over a number of weeks. Don't overdo it and expect instant results. If you push yourself too hard and too fast, you increase the risk of injury. I want long-term sustainability for you, not one weekend and done.

- Shoot for at least 30 to 60 minutes of moderate intensity physical activity, most days of the week.

- Forget "no pain, no gain." After starting a new activity, you will feel sore, but physical activity should make you feel exhilarated and exerted, not put you in severe pain. If you feel severe pain, especially any type of chest pain, stop and see a doctor immediately.

- Stay hydrated—drink water before, during, and after physical activity. Remember to warm up before you exercise and cool down at the end.

FOUR

NAIL YOUR HEALTH STATS

Hopefully by now you're warming up to the fact that you hold the keys to your own health. And by nailing your health stats, you'll use those keys to unlock the door of optimal wellness.

At first it can seem to be a very confusing, overwhelming process, but don't worry—I'll boil it down for you into a manageable set of tasks.

Actually, I'll make it really simple. For your optimal wellness, there are just five key sets of numbers I want you to track. If you do this, you will be doing wonders for your long-term health. Hey, you probably have at least a half-dozen passwords memorized, so why not remember a few more numbers when the payoff is so spectacular?

You should think of your body as the finest NASCAR-winning race car ever built. It is a masterpiece of engineering. It is capable of nearly miraculous performance. But it needs the best fuel, and it needs to be checked, pampered, and fine-tuned every few hundred laps!

I totally understand how tempting it is to skip your check-ups and doctor visits. I'm embarrassed to tell you this, but I recently went several years without getting a checkup. When you're in the hospital every day it's easy to justify blowing off a trip to see the doctor. Who wants to go to the doctor on their day off? Not me. But the fact is, getting your checkups will prevent illnesses and can even save your life.

I know some doctors who haven't had a proper physical exam in over a decade, and they have no idea what their key health stats are.

They could be ticking time bombs of disease ready to go off at any moment, and they haven't a clue—and they're doctors! Last year on our
show *The Doctors*, all four of us cohosts turned the tables on ourselves
by undergoing some crucial exams each one of us had been putting
off for too long. We took our lab coats off and put the hospital gowns
on. With the cameras rolling, I hopped on a treadmill and underwent
a cardiac stress test in the middle of our show. Given my history of
higher than normal blood pressure, plus the fact that I was having
some chest pain that I was attributing to a terrible case of bronchitis I
couldn't seem to kick, I figured this was an excellent idea.

A stress test determines the ability of the heart to handle the "stress"
caused by a controlled period of exercise. When under stress, your heart
requires more oxygen, and the stress test can reveal whether the heart
has enough oxygen or if the blood supply is reduced or compromised.
It can identify abnormalities that wouldn't be evident in a resting situation. The test is easy to take and widely available, so if you have risk
factors (such as high blood pressure, being a smoker, a family history
of heart disease, high cholesterol, diabetes, known heart disease) and
symptoms of heart disease (classic symptoms are chest pain and shortness of breath, but sometimes symptoms are much more subtle), it's a
good idea to discuss with your doctor whether you may need one.

Off came my shirt. The technician squeezed adhesive goop to my
chest, attached the monitors, and I got onto a treadmill set at a low
speed and a steep incline.

I was anxious. I figured I was in good physical shape, but this was
happening on national television, and I had no idea what data the
equipment would reveal. Believe me; I did not relish the possibility of
being called out as a hypocrite in front of millions of TV viewers!

I marched away on the treadmill, and soon felt a bit winded as I
climbed toward an 80 percent maximum heart rate. Minutes passed,
and finally the doctor who administered the test huddled up with the
technician around the machines to analyze the results, looking for
abnormalities in the data and images on the screens.

The Moment of Truth arrived, and . . . it turned out fine. Nothing out of the ordinary showed up. The doctor reported I had an above average level of fitness and my heart was in good shape.

Next, my colleague Dr. Lisa Masterson, an OB/GYN, got a mammogram on the air. For a woman, it's one of the most important, lifesaving tests of all.

A mammogram is a type of imaging that uses low-dose X-rays to examine the breast. The images help in the early detection and diagnosis of breast diseases in women. At the time of this writing, they are recommended by the American Cancer Society every year for women over forty and often earlier for women with a family history of breast cancer. It's the primary screening tool doctors have to detect stages of breast cancer. (See page 142 for special note on when to have a mammogram.)

This was an emotional experience for Lisa. Her mother died of breast cancer when Lisa was in medical school. "My mom was my best friend," she explained. "She raised me as a single mother." Lisa's mom inspired her to become a doctor. Dr. Lisa confessed to the audience that her family history made it emotionally difficult for her to get regular mammograms. "I'm embarrassed to say that I can't remember the last time I had a mammogram, even though I don't know how many times a day I tell every single one of my patients to get one!"

When I heard her say this, I thought, we're all human beings, we all get afraid.

She went in for the test, stepped up to the machine, and took a deep breath. She was anxious to get the results, as every woman is. But she was happy she got it done.

The results? Great news. The radiologist analyzed Lisa's mammogram and found everything was normal.

Then, plastic surgeon and reconstructive surgery expert Dr. Andrew Ordon bravely dropped his drawers and submitted himself for a televised prostate examination.

Now, that's real courage, I thought, as my cohost laughed and gave us the thumbs-up on the examining table where an ultrasonic probe was inserted into his rectum.

"I didn't get any Barry White music!" Dr. Drew wisecracked as ultrasound images of his prostate appeared on the screen for the world to see.

A prostate exam is an extremely important test for men. It's recommended for all men at normal risk starting at age fifty, African-American men starting at age forty, and age forty for men with a family history of prostate cancer (or younger, if recommended by a doctor), and for men who experience persistent difficulty urinating.

The exam is a test to screen for prostate cancer, which affects about one out of seven men. The purpose is to identify cancer early, when treatment can be most effective. The most common prostate exam is the digital rectal exam, or DRE, where the doctor inserts his or her gloved, lubricated finger into a man's rectum to feel the prostate gland and surrounding tissue. A PSA blood test is also used to measure prostate-specific antigens (PSA), a substance produced by the prostate gland. Elevated PSA levels may indicate prostate cancer or a noncancerous condition such as prostatitis, or an enlarged prostate. Drew was getting a more detailed ultrasound exam, because he had a history of both a high PSA and prostatitis.

The examining doctor spotted some cysts, or fluid-filled masses, in his prostate area, and also some calcification, signs of prostatitis that Dr. Drew was aware he had. The next step was for Dr. Drew to take images from the exam to his urologist, and for both to keep a regular eye on his PSA and the cysts to check for any deterioration, in which case a biopsy would be warranted.

Ultimately, the test revealed nothing to be alarmed about. But taking the test was an excellent move by Dr. Drew to stay on top of his health.

Things got trickier when it came to pediatrician Dr. Jim Sears, a man who has become both my on-air colleague and friend.

"For the last year or two, I've had a little blind spot in my eye," he confided to the audience. "I've ignored it, which is not the best thing to do." So we joined him as he went to get his eye tested. Needless to say he was apprehensive, and he braced himself in case the news was bad.

Ophthalmologist Dr. Sanford Chen performed a visual inspection of Dr. Jim's cornea, lens, iris, and pupil. Next, he performed a fluorescein angiogram test, which examines the microcirculation and integrity of the retinal blood vessels at the back of the eye. To do this, Dr. Chen injected dye into a vein in Jim's arm, which traveled into his eye in less than ten seconds. The dye illuminated sections of the retina that are otherwise not visible. This enabled Dr. Chen to see if Jim had a blockage in one of his blood vessels, or a stroke.

The result: "Good news and bad news," reported Dr. Chen.

"The good news is the fluorescein angiogram part of the test looked great. The blood flow was good, the circulation was fine. Your retina looks good. Interestingly, however, the color pictures that we took prior to giving you the dye were where we saw some abnormalities."

Dr. Chen concluded that Dr. Jim's optic nerve was abnormal, which could be caused by growths or lesions on his nerve.

"Doesn't sound good," Jim said as he absorbed the news.

"The most worrisome thing, of course, is a brain tumor," Dr. Chen said.

I was standing right next to Dr. Jim, and I could feel the palpable impact of those two words, things you never want to hear when talking with your doctor.

"That's what we always worry about when we see abnormal optic nerves," Dr. Chen said. "The chances of that are low, but the next step is getting an MRI, a CT scan of the brain, and an ultrasound of the optic nerve."

There was a happy ending to the story—Jim's follow-up tests found no brain tumor and no other problems. The blind spot Jim was experiencing was the result of a manageable congenital deformity.

When it was all over, Jim felt really good that he underwent the tests and finally got some answers.

For me, the lesson from our round of tests was crystal clear—I should never be afraid to "man up" and get tested, and I should do everything I can to nail my health stats.

The same thing goes for you, too: just "woman up" or "man up," and get it done. It's easier than you think!

As I've said, I love to cut through the clutter. When you work in an emergency room for a living, you pick up this habit quickly. The clock is ticking, medical crises erupt, and as a doctor you've got to figure out what the problem is and fix it, fast. To accomplish this, you push all extraneous information out of your brain and focus on solving the problem for the patient.

You can apply the same thinking to your health.

I'll explain in the following pages by giving you a rundown on the five health stats that can save your life—and one number that you always want to keep at absolute zero.

Key Stat #1

Get to a healthy weight by having a body mass index (BMI) of under 25, a waist size of under 35 inches for women and under 40 inches for men.

Your body mass index, or BMI, is one of your absolutely most critical health stats. Why? The higher your BMI is over a healthy weight, the higher your risks are for many chronic diseases. If you're at a healthy weight, however, you are optimizing your health in a huge way.

Measure your BMI right now. It's easy—just find your weight and height on the BMI chart below, which rounds off the numbers.

Drumroll, please.

Adult BMI Chart

BMI	19	20	21	22	23	24	25	26	27	28	29	30	31	32	33	34	35
Height							**Weight in Pounds**										
4'10"	91	96	100	105	110	115	119	124	129	134	138	143	148	153	158	162	167
4'11"	94	99	104	109	114	119	124	128	133	138	143	148	153	158	163	168	173
5'	97	102	107	112	118	123	128	133	138	143	148	153	158	163	168	174	179
5'1"	100	106	111	116	122	127	132	137	143	148	153	158	164	169	174	180	185
5'2"	104	109	115	120	126	131	136	142	147	153	158	164	169	175	180	186	191
5'3"	107	113	118	124	130	135	141	146	152	158	163	169	175	180	186	191	197
5'4"	110	116	122	128	134	140	145	151	157	163	169	174	180	186	192	197	204
5'5"	114	120	123	132	138	144	150	156	162	168	174	180	186	192	198	204	210
5'6"	118	124	130	136	142	148	155	161	167	173	179	186	192	198	204	210	216
5'7"	121	127	134	140	146	153	159	166	172	178	185	191	198	204	211	217	223
5'8"	125	131	138	144	151	158	164	171	177	184	190	197	203	210	216	223	230
5'9"	128	135	142	149	155	162	169	176	182	189	196	203	209	216	223	230	236
5'10"	132	139	146	153	160	167	174	181	188	195	202	209	216	222	229	236	243
5'11"	136	143	150	157	165	172	179	186	193	200	208	215	222	229	236	243	250
6'	140	147	154	162	169	177	184	191	199	206	213	221	228	235	242	250	258
6'1"	144	151	159	166	174	182	189	197	204	212	219	227	235	242	250	257	265
6'2"	148	155	163	171	179	186	194	202	210	218	225	233	241	249	256	264	272
6'3"	152	160	168	176	184	192	200	208	216	224	232	240	248	256	264	272	279
	Healthy Weight						Overweight					Obese					

Note: You can also calculate your BMI online at www.nhlbisupport.com/bmi or www
.cdc.gov/healthyweight/assessing/bmi/index.html. Also, *The Doctors* has a link from our
website, www.thedoctorstv.com. Just type in a search for BMI calculator. And be sure to
weigh yourself without shoes or clothes on!

Okay, how did you do?

A BMI of 18.5 to 24.9 is considered healthy. Below that is considered underweight, in which case you should talk to your doctor about creating a plan for gaining weight. A BMI of 25 to 29.9 is considered overweight, which carries increased health risks; and a BMI of 30 or more is considered obese, which carries even more severe health risks. As I discussed in earlier chapters, extra weight puts you at greater risk of a host of health problems, including cardiovascular diseases, hypertension, dyslipidemia, type 2 diabetes, some forms of cancer, and other illnesses. And the risk increases with more and more weight.

I weigh 195 pounds. I'm also 6 foot 4 inches tall, so I'm too tall for the chart above! So I just went to our website, www.thedoctorstv .com, searched for BMI calculator, loaded in the numbers, and saw that my BMI is 23.7, which puts me in the healthy weight category. You definitely want to be in the healthy weight zone. If you aren't there, getting there should be a top health priority.

It's worth repeating: you want your BMI to be below 25.

The body mass index is a good measurement used by many health professionals, but it's not perfect. It may, for example, overestimate body fat for athletes and others with a muscular build, and it may underestimate body fat in older people and others who have lost muscle mass. Essentially, BMI is a screening tool that can be used to spark further discussion and assessment by you and your doctor.

The second way of measuring how close you are to a healthy weight is really simple—by measuring your waist. This measurement alone doesn't determine if you are overweight, but it does signal if you've got too much abdominal fat, which can elevate risks to your health like high blood pressure, blood sugar, cholesterol, and triglycerides. Abdominal fat, which is also known as belly fat and visceral fat, is considered more harmful than subcutaneous fat, which collects more around the hips, butt, and limbs. The bottom line—a beer belly or potbelly is extra hazardous to your health!

If you're a woman, you want your waist to measure 35 inches or less—preferably less. If you're a man, you want your waist to measure 40 inches or less—preferably less. According to the research, these numbers are a major threshold, above which health risks increase measurably.

There is a small but growing "fat acceptance" campaign in this country that's being promoted by some activists. They argue that our culture places too much emphasis on thinness, demonizes overweight and obese people, and overstates the risks of excess weight. Furthermore, they assert that people can and should be able to become healthy at any size.

I totally agree with some of their points. Nobody, especially young people, should ever be subjected to ridicule for their weight, and our media and culture must do a better job of respecting, showcasing, and celebrating people of all shapes and sizes. Also, some research suggests that carrying a bit of extra weight—for example, if you were at the lowest end of the overweight category on the BMI chart—isn't so terrible as long as you're being active and that even a little weight loss and extra physical activity can measurably improve health status in overweight and obese people. My mind is always open to research being debated, criticized, and improved.

But it's important to reiterate that one of the most critical medical facts you should know is that healthy eating and regular physical activity are excellent strategies for you to strive toward a healthy body weight—and a healthy body weight is one of the keys to optimal heath. "Virtually everyone who is overweight would be better off at a lower weight," Dr. Walter Willett, chairman of the nutrition department at the Harvard School of Public Health, said in the July 31, 2009 edition of *Time.* "There's been this misconception, fostered by the weight-is-beautiful groups, that weight doesn't matter. But the data are clear."

According to the National Institutes of Health (NIH), a highly respected U.S. government research body, most studies show an increase in mortality rates associated with obesity, and most of the extra risk is due to cardiovascular causes. Obesity is associated with some 112,000 excess deaths every year in the U.S. population.

If you are overweight or obese, you may be at increased risk for developing one or more of a witches' brew of health problems. It is a long and really frightening list. It's a list you want to stay away from. It includes: type 2 diabetes, coronary heart disease and stroke, metabolic syndrome, certain types of cancer, sleep apnea, osteoarthritis, gallbladder disease, fatty liver disease, fertility and pregnancy complications, surgical complications, gout, Alzheimer's disease, erectile dysfunction, and even psychological disorders like depression.

But according to the National Institutes of Health, there's also some great news:

How a Healthy Weight Optimizes Your Health

- A healthy weight reduces your risk for type 2 diabetes. More than 85 percent of people with type 2 diabetes are overweight. The Diabetes Prevention Program, a large clinical study sponsored by the National Institutes of Health, found that losing just 5 to 7 percent of your body weight and doing moderate-intensity exercise for 30 minutes a day, 5 days a week, may prevent or delay the onset of type 2 diabetes.

- A healthy weight reduces your risk for coronary heart disease and stroke. Coronary heart disease is the leading cause of death in the United States, and stroke is the third leading cause. Losing 5 to 10 percent of your weight will significantly lower your chances for developing coronary heart disease or having a stroke. If you weigh 200 pounds, this means losing as little as 10 pounds.

- A healthy weight reduces your risk for metabolic syndrome. The metabolic syndrome is a group of obesity-related risk factors for coronary heart disease and diabetes. A person with metabolic syndrome has approximately twice the risk for coronary heart disease and five times the risk for type 2 diabetes. It is estimated that 27 percent of American adults have the metabolic syndrome.

- A healthy weight reduces your risk for cancer. Being overweight increases the risk of developing several types of cancer, including cancers of the colon, esophagus, and kidney. Carrying extra pounds is also linked with uterine and postmenopausal breast cancer in women. Avoiding weight gain prevents a rise in cancer risk. Healthy eating and good physical activity habits lower cancer risk. Weight loss may also lower your risk.

Key Stat #2

Blood pressure: Keep it at or below 120 over 80.

It is very easy to get high blood pressure. It happened to me, just by eating everyday processed foods with too much added sodium.

Blood pressure is the force with which your blood pushes against your arterial walls in your bloodstream. High blood pressure can increase your risk for a blockage of a narrowed artery or trigger a break in a weakened blood vessel, either of which can cause a stroke. If it's too high, over time, it can also increase your risk for heart attacks, kidney failure, and death.

High blood pressure is a silent killer. Almost one in three American adults have high blood pressure, and many of them don't even know it. High blood pressure is particularly insidious because it creeps up on you quietly with no symptoms and no warning signs. Meanwhile, it puts a dangerous strain on the heart, forcing it to work too hard. Unfortunately, high blood pressure, also known as hypertension, is a condition that many people in the U.S. will have at some point in their lives, especially as they get into middle age. People at extra risk for developing high blood pressure include African Americans, people with a family history of high blood pressure, and overweight people.

Blood pressure is measured in milligrams of mercury (mm Hg). High blood pressure is defined as systolic pressure of 140 mm Hg or more, and diastolic pressure of 90 mm Hg or more. Prehypertension, which also needs to be monitored carefully, is a systolic pressure of 120 to 139 mm Hg or a diastolic pressure of 80 to 89 mm Hg. The higher your blood pressure numbers, the higher the risk to your health.

For optimal wellness, you want your blood pressure numbers to be at or below 120 over 80.

I recently checked my blood pressure on our TV show. I was happy to see it in a good healthy range—119 over 67.

There's only one good way to track your blood pressure, and that's to get it checked regularly at a doctor's office or other medical facility. Having said that, according to the National Institutes of Health, "Some people experience high blood pressure only when they visit the doctor's office." This effect is called "white-coat hypertension." It occurs when patients get especially nervous or stressed in the presence of the doctor. If your doctor thinks this might be happening, he or she can ask you to monitor your blood pressure at home, or by using a machine called an ambulatory blood pressure monitor, which can take sample readings over a one-day period.

The good news is that there are a number of effective medicines to help control blood pressure, and important things you can do, too. Here are tips on how to control your blood pressure, according to the American Heart Association and other experts:

- Get to a healthy weight.

- Eat a diet rich in fruits, vegetables, and whole-grain, high-fiber products, and low in saturated fat, trans fat, cholesterol, and sodium.

- Be more physically active—exercise can lower blood pressure as much as 10 points.

- Limit alcohol to no more than one drink per day for women or two drinks a day for men.

- Take medications as instructed by your doctor, and follow the directions.

- Get enough sleep—too little can increase your blood pressure.

- Know what your blood pressure should be and work to keep it at that level.

- Learn how to control stress in your life; taking a few deep breaths during stressful times of the day can make a big difference. When I feel anxious or acutely stressed and I don't have time for exercise (which is the best stress buster I know), I take a slow, deep breath, hold it for two seconds, and slowly exhale while counting to ten. I can almost feel my blood pressure drop!

Key Stat #3

Cholesterol: Get your total cholesterol under 200. Get your LDL below 130 if you're at intermediate risk for heart disease. Get your HDL checked as often as your doctor advises if you're a woman over fifty years old or a man over forty years old. Get your triglycerides to under 150.

Cholesterol is an essential fatty substance in your bloodstream that helps keep you healthy. But too much cholesterol in the blood can lead to atherosclerosis, coronary artery disease, stroke, heart attack, or death. How much we have is influenced by genetics, by the foods we eat, and by how active we are.

High-density lipoprotein, or HDL, is called "good" cholesterol because it pulls the bad cholesterol out of your system, and higher levels of HDL protect the heart.

Low-density lipoprotein, or LDL, is infamously called "bad" cholesterol since it helps lead to arteries blocking up with plaque, which can lead to heart attack and stroke. Data suggest that people who have more "small dense" LDL cholesterol may be at an even higher risk. In essence, smaller LDL particles may be the most dangerous. Stay tuned through your doctor for the latest updates on all these numbers.

Almost half of adult Americans have unhealthy levels of cholesterol, and a big reason is that they're eating too much saturated fat from animal products and processed foods. Dietary cholesterol can also contribute to the problems of too much cholesterol in your blood, but to a lesser degree than saturated fat. Can you eat eggs as part of a healthy diet? Sure. Just remember it's a question of balance. Remember the Eat to Savor Life target of less than 300 milligrams of cholesterol a day for people with normal LDL ("bad") cholesterol levels? One egg has around 213 milligrams of dietary cholesterol. So if you know your cholesterol levels are already high, you've got to balance things out.

Have your cholesterol checked regularly by your doctor with a simple blood test. Here are targets for your key cholesterol stats, recommended by health authorities:

Your Cholesterol Scorecard	
The stats you want:	
Total Cholesterol: The lower the better. Less than 200 mg/dL*	
LDL ("Bad") Cholesterol: The lower the better. Note: There are different goals for each level of risk for heart disease	
People who are at low risk for heart disease	Less than 160 mg/dL
People at intermediate risk for heart disease	Less than 130 mg/dL
People at high risk for heart disease including those who have heart disease or diabetes	Less than 100 mg/dL
People at very high risk for heart disease	Less than 70 mg/dL
HDL ("Good") Cholesterol: The higher the better.	
Women	50 mg/dL or higher
Men	40 mg/dL or higher
TRIGLYCERIDES: The lower the better. 10 to 150 mg/dL	

*milligrams per deciliter (mg/dL) of blood.

You can improve your stats on your own by Eating to Savor Life and treating yourself to a Daily Physical Vacation. According to the American Heart Association and other authorities, here are some of the most important tips to improve your cholesterol and triglyceride levels and help prevent heart disease and heart attack:

- Eat a heart-healthy diet with plenty of fiber-rich fruits and vegetables.

- Minimize saturated fats, trans fats, and dietary cholesterol in your diet.

- Substitute fish high in omega-3 fatty acids in place of meats high in saturated fat like hamburger meat. Fatty fish like mackerel, lake trout, herring, sardines, and salmon are high in omega-3 fatty acids.

- Exercise regularly, which helps raise HDL ("good") cholesterol.

- Work toward a healthy body weight.

- Quit smoking.

- Reduce your intake of alcohol considerably. Too much alcohol can lead to large changes in plasma triglyceride levels.

- Get periodic health checkups and cholesterol screenings.

- Follow the National Cholesterol Education Program (NCEP) guidelines for detection of high cholesterol: Everyone age twenty and older should have a fasting lipoprotein profile test every five years. This test is done after a nine- to twelve-hour fast without food, liquids, or pills. It measures total cholesterol, LDL, HDL, and triglycerides. Adults should be screened more often if they have unfavorable cholesterol numbers and/or if they have other cardiac risk factors.

- Work with your doctor to improve your cholesterol numbers. He or she may suggest medication that will help, such as statins.

Key Stat #4

Get your fasting glucose under 100.

Blood glucose, or blood sugar, is a primary source of energy for your body's cells. It comes from what we eat and drink. Your body needs it to run properly. But health risks rise when your blood glucose registers outside the normal levels.

High blood sugar is like high blood pressure. It's largely silent initially but over time, it leads not just to increased heart attack risk but also to kidney failure, blindness, life and limb threatening infections, and extremity numbness. And, in most instances, it is all preventable.

This stat is very simple and straightforward. You want your fasting glucose score to be under 100 mg/dL. If your score is over that number, talk to your doctor about lifestyle improvements you can put into action and medication you can consider to get it under control.

If your doctor thinks you might have diabetes or prediabetes, he or she may suggest a test of your blood or urine to measure glucose, which is sugar your body uses for energy. The test is used to screen for and diagnose diabetes.

The test can be a good idea if you're forty-five years of age or older, especially if you have a BMI of 25 or over (23 or over for Asian Americans) and/or you have other risk factors for diabetes like a family history of the condition.

Key Stat #5

Calculate your personal calorie target—and hit the bull's-eye with healthy eating and physical activity.

Okay, if a healthy body weight is so crucial to our health, how, then, can we get there? The secret to a healthy weight is actually quite simple. According to the NIH, it's "what and how much you eat and how much physical activity you do during the whole day that determines whether you gain, lose, or maintain your weight."

If you want to get to a healthy weight, there's an easy-to-calculate familiar formula you need to burn into your brain: calories in minus calories out. Take how many calories you consume in the form of food and beverages, and subtract the calories burned off during the physical activity you engage in. If the two numbers are equal, your weight stays the same.

ALL YOU EVER NEED TO KNOW ABOUT CALORIES
(thanks to the website MyPyramid.gov)

- A calorie is defined as a unit of energy supplied by food. A calorie is a calorie regardless of its source. Whether you're eating carbohydrates, fats, or proteins, all of them contain calories. If your diet focus is on reducing any one of these groups alone, you're missing the bigger picture.

- When it comes to maintaining a healthy weight for a lifetime, the bottom line is calories count! Weight management is all about balance—balancing the number of calories you consume with the number of calories your body burns off.

- Caloric balance is like a scale. To remain in balance and maintain your body weight, the calories consumed (from foods and beverages) must be balanced by the calories used (in normal body functions, daily activities, and exercise).

- To lose weight, calories in should be less than calories out.

- To gain weight, calories in should be more than calories out.

That sounds easy, but how do we make it work in the real world? How are we supposed to track every move we make and every calorie we consume?

My answer is you don't need to bother.

Some people do well with weight loss by relentlessly counting calories. If you can do it and find it works for you, that's fantastic. It's certainly a great way to figure out your daily calorie average and an excellent way to start a lifestyle change. Weight Watchers, a widely respected plan, is based on carefully keeping track of calories, and it has helped millions of people work toward a healthy weight. But personally, I take a more relaxed approach that I'll call being calorie-savvy, rather than calorie-obsessed, which for me would take up too much time. I check food labels and restaurant nutritional information for calorie counts so I have a rough idea of how many calories I'm taking in. I eat healthy and I work out regularly. On top of that, I'm lucky to have a very active job in the ER where I'm on my feet and moving around almost nonstop. The result: over time, I've come to instinctively get a day-to-day feel for reaching my calorie target, or the magic number of calories in and calories out I need to hit every day, on average, to stay in the healthy weight zone.

America's weight problem can be boiled down to just two numbers. The average American is consuming roughly 3,800 calories a day, when the number for many people should be closer to roughly 2,000 to 2,800. When you combine this with our too-sedentary lifestyles in which technology has largely removed the need for us to move anywhere, the result is a massive national weight imbalance and a rampant epidemic of obesity and related illnesses. Human beings are simply not engineered to carry this calorie overload without getting sick. Our bodies don't know what to do with all the extra weight, so it gets stored as excess fat, and we get diabetes, heart disease, and all the rest.

The good news is there is an easy way for you to figure out what your daily personal calorie target should be. The MyPyramid.gov website has an excellent feature called MyPyramid Plan, www.mypyramid.gov/mypyramid/index.aspx, where you can type in five key pieces of information, and calculate an estimate of how many calories you should be taking in each day, or what I call your Personal Calorie Target. The number varies depending on your age, gender, genetics, weight, activity level, and whether you're trying to gain, maintain, or lose weight.

The website gives you an instant healthy eating plan based on your ideal daily calorie pattern. You can use the plan not as a rigid therapeutic "bible" to slavishly adhere to, but as a good guideline of goals and patterns to work toward day to day and week to week.

The calorie number generated by the website, or what I call Your Personal Calorie Target, is a key health stat you should know and keep in the back of your mind. Once you know it, you can do a much better job of being calorie-conscious and calorie responsible, and you can more clearly see the big picture of how you can take charge of your body and your habits and work toward the goal of a healthy weight.

Take me, for example. I am a thirty-eight-year-old male who is six feet four inches tall, weighs 195 pounds, and does moderate-to-vigorous physical activity for more than sixty minutes a day. I loaded those numbers into the MyPyramid Plan website, and it generated for me a 3,200-calories-a-day food pattern for me.

Here are examples of other sample Personal Calorie Targets, based on the MyPyramid Plan website. Remember, these are averages and estimates, not necessarily precise for every person. Your calorie needs can be more or less than the averages, so check your weight regularly and if you see unwanted weight gain or loss, consult with your doctor.

Sample Personal Calorie Targets

(courtesy of www.mypyramid.gov)

- A twenty-six-year-old female who is five feet two inches tall, weighs 140 pounds (which is above the healthy weight range for this height), and is physically active for more than 60 minutes a day: a 2,200 calorie food pattern, to gradually move to a healthier weight.

- A thirty-eight-year old female who is 5 feet 6 inches tall, weighs 135 pounds, and is physically active 30 to 60 minutes a day: a 2,200 calorie food pattern, to stay in the healthy weight range.

- A forty-year-old female who is 5 feet 7 inches tall, weighs 160 pounds (which is above the healthy weight range for this height), and is physically active less than 30 minutes a day: an 1,800 calorie food pattern, to gradually move to a healthier weight.

- A forty-five-year-old male who is 5 feet 11 inches tall, weighs 175 pounds, and is physically active 30 to 60 minutes a day: a 2,800 calorie food pattern, to stay in the healthy weight range.

- A fifty-two-year-old male who is 5 feet 9 inches tall, weighs 200 pounds (which is above the healthy weight range for this height), and is physically active less than 30 minutes a day: a 2,200 calorie food pattern, to gradually move to a healthier weight.

Note: This site defines physical activity as "the amount of moderate or vigorous activity (such as brisk walking, jogging, biking, aerobics, or yardwork) you do in addition to your normal daily routine, most days."

What's your Personal Calorie Target? Find out now!

Don't forget that a huge key to optimal wellness is not just how many calories you eat/drink and burn off every day, but also the quality of the calories you take in.

You want those calories to reflect the Eat to Savor Life philosophy by being based largely on many different kinds of whole veggies and fruit; whole grains; and healthy foods like fish, nuts, and beans—and less sodium, bad fats, added sugars, and processed foods.

The One Stat You Must Always Keep at Absolute Zero

I'm going to tell you a true horror story. It's called smoking. There is nothing more deadly and deleterious to your health.

Over 43 million Americans smoke cigarettes, including 20 percent of all adults, and an equal percentage of high school students. And it is going to kill millions of them.

Let's be very clear about this—smoking doesn't just kill you. That's bad enough, but it's actually worse. Smoking, in many cases, literally tortures you to death over the course of many agonizing years of medical torment. It creates a flesh-and-blood living hell for millions of people. As a doctor, I see no need to pull punches or sugarcoat the truth when it comes to smoking. It literally creates a kind of nightmare on Earth. In the emergency room, I regularly see victims of the self-inflicted horrors of tobacco.

If you think smoking is sexy, or fun, or enjoyable, come spend a day in the ER with me taking care of long-term smokers. Take a look at the physical agony that smoking has inflicted on them and their families.

Peek in on the lady in Room 5 who is suffering from chronic obstructive pulmonary disease, or COPD, struggling for every breath, connected to an oxygen tank. She can only speak in one- or two-word sentences. How did she land in the emergency room? She smokes cigarettes.

There's a woman in Room 1 who had to have her left foot amputated due to claudication as a result of peripheral vascular disease caused by smoking.

Have a look at the man in the operating room who just suffered a massive heart attack at age fifty-one. He's been smoking for thirty years. He will not see his kids graduate from high school. He's going to die in eight minutes.

And there's a forty-year-old in Room 3, a wife and mother of four who looks like an unhealthy sixty-year-old because she's spent her entire adult life smoking cigarettes. Ask them if they had it to do all over again—would they smoke?

These are real people I've seen, typical of people I see all the time. As their ER doctor, I tell them things like this: "You came here today because your asthma has gotten much worse, but the real reason you came here today was for me to say you need to quit smoking right now. The best thing I can do for you today is to tell you to stop smoking. You just may add ten to twenty years to your life." Maybe only one out of ten people I say that to will actually quit, but that's better than nothing.

Smokers can't fool me. As a doctor, I can tell within five seconds of meeting you if you're a long-term smoker. Your skin looks different. You get fine lines on your face. When I listen to you breathe I'll hear the faint wheezing from what I call a "smoker's lung," which is the first step toward developing COPD.

We have a president of the United States who smoked cigarettes for years. That's how powerful the addiction is. President Obama has readily admitted how difficult it is to stop smoking. The cigarette companies have taken an already addictive substance, the nicotine in tobacco, and made it even more addictive. It is an overwhelmingly powerful addiction, and the result is you have some of the world's most intelligent and high-functioning people who keep smoking, despite the fact that they know it will probably kill them. Not being able to quit is not a sign of any lack of intelligence—it's a sign of how incredibly addictive smoking is. I've tried cigarettes before, so I know the power that nicotine can have flowing through your system.

I paid a visit to New York City recently and I simply could not believe how many people were crowded around the entrances of office buildings at midday, puffing away. It completely blows my mind that anyone would ever smoke throughout their lives, when the dangers are so well-known, and so open-and-shut. Smoking is an excellent, scientifically proven way of committing suicide.

I'll spare you the most gruesome details, but consider these stark, flesh-and-blood facts:

- Smoking kills 440,000 smokers every year in the U.S. according to the American Cancer Society, and kills nearly 50,000 nonsmokers every year who are exposed to tobacco smoke. It is the most preventable cause of premature death in our society.

- Smoking may chop over thirteen years off the life of the average smoker.

- The vast majority of people who smoke are going to be killed by smoking.

- Every puff of cigarette smoke contains thousands of chemicals that can hurt almost every organ in the body. Smoking either causes or increases the risk of heart disease, aneurysms, bronchitis, emphysema, stroke, infertility, early menopause, and a great many different cancers, including cancers of the lung, colon and rectum, oral cavity, nasal cavities and nasal sinuses, pharynx, larynx, esophagus, stomach, pancreas, liver, bladder, kidney, uterine, cervix, and myeloid leukemia.

- Smoking is also linked to gum disease, cataracts, bone thinning, hip fractures, peptic ulcers, erectile dysfunction, macular degeneration, and peripheral vascular disease, and it makes asthma and any bout with pneumonia worse.

- Secondhand smoke causes up to 300,000 cases of lower respiratory tract infections in children under eighteen months of age in the United States each year.

There's only one simple number you need to keep in mind when it comes to smoking: absolute zero.

If you smoke, the single most important thing you can do for your health is to quit right away. The good news is, if you quit, much of the damage to your body can be slowed, stopped, or even reversed. But you must realize that a smoke-free life is crucial to your health, and eliminate all tobacco products from your life immediately.

Those are my doctor's orders!

It's tough to quit, no doubt. Nicotine is physically addictive and emotionally very hard to shake. It can take you several tries before you succeed. But, boy, is it worth it! Quitting smoking has major health benefits that start right away. This is true for people who already have smoking-related disease as well as those who don't.

Sure, some people put on a bit of weight after quitting, but it's usually less than ten pounds, and the health benefits of stopping smoking vastly outweigh any small, temporary weight gain. And once you quit, you may feel it's easier to exercise and eat healthier as part of your new healthy life.

According to the Surgeon General and the Department of Health and Human Services, here are some of the powerful ways you can optimize your health when you cut out tobacco.

- Twenty minutes after quitting: your heart rate and blood pressure drops.

- Twelve hours after quitting: the carbon monoxide level in your blood drops to normal.

- Two weeks to three months after quitting: your circulation improves and your lung function increases.

- One to nine months after quitting: coughing and shortness of breath decrease; cilia (tiny hairlike structures that move mucus out of the lungs) regain normal function in the lungs, increasing the ability to handle mucus, clean the lungs, and reduce the risk of infection.

- One year after quitting: the excess risk of coronary heart disease is half that of before.

- Five years after quitting: your stroke risk may be reduced to that of a nonsmoker.

- Ten years after quitting: the lung cancer death rate is about half that of a continuing smoker's. The risk of cancer of the mouth, throat, esophagus, bladder, cervix, and pancreas decrease.

- Fifteen years after quitting: the risk of coronary heart disease is that of a nonsmoker's.

- Former smokers live longer than people who keep smoking. For example, people who quit smoking before age fifty have one half the risk of dying in the next fifteen years compared with people who keep smoking.

- Quitting smoking lowers the risk of lung cancer, other cancers, heart attack, stroke, and chronic lung diseases such as emphysema and chronic bronchitis.

- Women who stop smoking before they get pregnant reduce their risk of having a low birth-weight baby to that of women who never smoked. Even women who quit during the first three to four months of pregnancy have much healthier babies than those who keep smoking.

It is absolutely never too late to stop smoking. If you quit in your twenties or thirties, you can avoid most of the risk. But even if you quit in your forties or fifties, you can still greatly decrease your risk for premature death.

People quit in many ways—cold turkey on their own, or with the help of medications, or counseling, or by setting a personal Quit Day. Nicotine replacement products like patches, gums, lozenges, and nasal sprays can help you fight off cravings. Medications like bupropion SR or varenicline, used in conjunction with nicotine replacement, can double the chances of quitting. And lower tar and lower nicotine cigarettes are not the solution—they provide no clear health benefit. Ask your doctor for more information and for help. And remember, you can do it. You are better and stronger than the tobacco, and like millions of others who have successfully quit, you can, too. It isn't easy, but you really can do it. Commit right now. Don't give up. Even if it takes you a couple of attempts, you can do it!

If you've attempted to quit but couldn't after a few tries, don't get discouraged—think of it as good practice for the real thing!

A couple came up to me in the hospital a month ago and told me they recognized me from TV and wanted to thank me. "For what?" I asked. "You inspired us to live healthier lives because of what you keep saying on the show," they replied. They decided to eat much healthier and start exercising regularly. They did it together as husband and wife, as a team. And the best part was when they told me this: "We both quit smoking."

That was a very good day for me.

Dr. Stork's Tip for Smokers and Other Tobacco Users: Call 1-800-QuitNow.

I refer all my smoking patients to this national quit line. It's an excellent free service provided by the National Institutes of Health and the National Cancer Institute to help people stop smoking or quit other forms of tobacco use.

When you call 1-800-QuitNow, you'll have access to many different types of cessation information and services, including free advice from a counselor, a personalized quit plan and self-help materials, social support and coping strategies to help you deal with cravings, and the latest information about cessation medications that can help you quit.

For more tips and resources on how to quit, go to www.smokefree .gov and click on Quit Smoking Today!

THE HEALTH TESTS YOU SHOULD TAKE

A powerful, essential step to help you nail your stats is to get the right screening tests, so you and your doctor can spot problems early, when they're easier to treat. Below is a rundown of the most important tests recommended by experts from the U.S. Preventive Services Task Force. Talk to your doctor about which ones apply to you, and when and how often you should be tested. He or she may suggest other tests as well.

For Women

- **Obesity:** Have your body mass index (BMI) calculated to screen for obesity. (BMI is a measure of body fat based on height and weight.) You can also find your own BMI with the BMI calculator from the National Heart, Lung, and Blood Institute at: www.nhlbisupport.com/bmi/

- **Breast Cancer:** Have a mammogram every one to two years starting at age forty or fifty, depending on your doctor's opinion. There is a dispute among the experts over whether to start at age forty or fifty—the American Cancer Society recommends forty, and the U.S. Preventive Services Task Force recommends fifty. Ask your doctor how the risks and benefits apply specifically to you and at what age you should start routine screening.

- **Cervical Cancer:** Have a Pap smear every one to three years if you:

  - Have ever been sexually active.

  - Are between the ages of twenty-one and sixty-five.

- **High Cholesterol:** Have your cholesterol checked regularly starting at age forty-five. (Some experts suggest starting as early as twenty.) If you are younger than forty-five, talk to your doctor about whether you need to have your cholesterol checked if:

  - You have diabetes.

  - You have high blood pressure.

  - Heart disease runs in your family.

  - You smoke.

- **High Blood Pressure:** Have your blood pressure checked at least every two years. High blood pressure is 140/90 or higher.

- **Colorectal Cancer:** Have a test for colorectal cancer starting at age fifty. Your doctor can help you decide which test is right for you. If you have a family history of colorectal cancer, you may need to be screened earlier.

- **Diabetes:** Have a test for diabetes if you have high blood pressure or high cholesterol.

- **Depression:** Your emotional health is as important as your physical health. If you have felt "down," sad, or hopeless over the last two weeks or have felt little interest or pleasure in doing things, you may be depressed. Talk to your doctor about being screened for depression.

- **Osteoporosis (thinning of the bones):** Have a bone density test, also called a densitometry or DXA scan, beginning at age sixty-five to screen for osteoporosis. If you are between the ages of sixty and sixty-four and weigh 154 pounds or less, talk to your doctor about being tested.

- **Chlamydia and Other Sexually Transmitted Infections:** Have a test for chlamydia if you are twenty-five or younger and sexually active. If you are older, talk to your doctor about being tested. Also ask whether you should be tested for other sexually transmitted diseases.

- **HIV:** Have a test to screen for HIV infection if you:

  - Have had unprotected sex with multiple partners.

  - Are pregnant.

  - Have used or now use injection drugs.

  - Exchange sex for money or drugs or have sex partners who do.

  - Have past or present sex partners who are HIV infected, are bisexual, or use injection drugs.

  - Are being treated for sexually transmitted diseases.

  - Had a blood transfusion between 1978 and 1985.

- **Should You Take Medicines to Prevent Disease?**

  - **Hormones:** Do not take hormones to prevent disease. Talk to your doctor if you need relief from the symptoms of menopause.

■ **Breast Cancer Drugs:** If your mother, sister, or daughter has had breast cancer, talk to your doctor about the risks and benefits of taking medicines to prevent breast cancer.

■ **Aspirin:** Ask your doctor about taking aspirin to prevent heart disease if you are:

- ◆ Older than forty-five

- ◆ Younger than forty-five and:

  - • Have high blood pressure.

  - • Have high cholesterol.

  - • Have diabetes.

  - • Smoke.

■ **Immunizations:** To stay up-to-date with your immunizations:

- ◆ Have a flu shot every year starting at age fifty. If you are younger than fifty, ask your doctor whether you need a flu shot.

- ◆ Get a pneumonia vaccine once you turn sixty-five. If you are younger, ask your doctor whether you need a pneumonia shot.

The Centers for Disease Control and Prevention provide more information on immunizations at: http://www.cdc.gov/vaccines/recs/schedules/adult-schedule.htm.

Women's Screening Test Checklist

Take this checklist with you to your doctor's office. Write down the last date that you have had any of the tests below. Talk to your doctor about your test results and write down what he or she says here. Ask when you should have the test next, and write down the month and year. If you think of questions for the doctor, write them down and bring them to your next visit.

Test	Last Test (mo/yr)	Results	Next Test Due (mo/yr)	Questions for the Doctor
Weight (BMI)				
Cholesterol Total:				
HDL ("good"):				
LDL ("bad"):				

Test	Last Test (mo/yr)	Results	Next Test Due (mo/yr)	Questions for the Doctor
Blood pressure				
Mammogram				
Pap smear				
Colorectal cancer				

Test	Last Test (mo/yr)	Results	Next Test Due (mo/yr)	Questions for the Doctor
Diabetes				
Sexually transmitted infections				
HIV infection				
Bone density				

Source: Adapted from U.S. Preventive Services Task Force

For Men

- **Obesity:** Have your body mass index (BMI) calculated to screen for obesity. (BMI is a measure of body fat based on height and weight.) You can also find your own BMI with the BMI calculator from the National Heart, Lung, and Blood Institute at: www.nhlbisupport.com/bmi/.

- **High Cholesterol:** Have your cholesterol checked regularly starting at age thirty-five. (Some experts suggest starting as early as twenty.) If you are younger than thirty-five, talk to your doctor about whether to have your cholesterol checked if:

  - You have diabetes.

  - You have high blood pressure.

  - Heart disease runs in your family.

  - You smoke.

- **High Blood Pressure:** Have your blood pressure checked at least every two years. High blood pressure is 140/90 or higher.

- **Colorectal Cancer:** Have a test for colorectal cancer starting at age fifty. Your doctor can help you decide which test is right for you. If you have a family history of colorectal cancer, you may need to be screened earlier.

- **Diabetes:** Have a test for diabetes if you have high blood pressure or high cholesterol.

- **Depression:** Your emotional health is as important as your physical health. If you have felt "down," sad, or hopeless over the last two weeks or have felt little interest or pleasure in doing things, you may be depressed. Talk to your doctor about being screened for depression.

- **Sexually Transmitted Infections:** Talk to your doctor to see whether you should be tested for gonorrhea, syphilis, chlamydia, or other sexually transmitted infections.

- **HIV:** Talk to your doctor about HIV screening if you:

  - Have had sex with men since 1975.

  - Have had unprotected sex with multiple partners.

  - Have used or now use injection drugs.

  - Exchange sex for money or drugs or have sex partners who do.

  - Have past or present sex partners who are HIV infected, are bisexual, or use injection drugs.

  - Are being treated for sexually transmitted diseases.

  - Had a blood transfusion between 1978 and 1985.

- **Abdominal Aortic Aneurysm.** If you are between the ages of sixty-five and seventy-five and have ever smoked (100 or more cigarettes during your lifetime), you need to be screened once for abdominal aortic aneurysm, which is an abnormally large or swollen blood vessel in your abdomen.

- **Should You Take Medicines to Prevent Disease?**

  - **Aspirin:** Ask your doctor about taking aspirin to prevent heart disease if you are:

    - Older than forty-five.

    - Younger than forty-five and:

- Have high blood pressure.

- Have high cholesterol.

- Have diabetes.

- Smoke.

■ **Immunizations:** Stay up-to-date with your immunizations:

♦ Have a flu shot every year starting at age fifty. If you are younger than fifty, ask your doctor whether you need a flu shot.

♦ Have a pneumonia shot once after you turn sixty-five. If you are younger, ask your doctor whether you need a pneumonia shot.

The Centers for Disease Control and Prevention provide more information on immunizations at: http://www.cdc.gov/vaccines/recs/ schedules/adult-schedule.htm.

Men's Screening Test Checklist

Take this checklist with you to your doctor's office. Write down the last date you had any of the tests below. Talk to your doctor about your test results and write down what he or she says here. Ask when you should have the test next. Write down the month and year. If you think of questions for the doctor, write them down and bring them to your next visit.

Test	Last Test (mo/yr)	Results	Next Test Due (mo/yr)	Questions for the Doctor
Weight (BMI)				
Cholesterol Total:				
HDL (good):				

Test	Last Test (mo/yr)	Results	Next Test Due (mo/yr)	Questions for the Doctor
LDL (bad):				
Blood pressure				
Colorectal cancer				
Diabetes				

Test	Last Test (mo/yr)	Results	Next Test Due (mo/yr)	Questions for the Doctor
Sexually transmitted diseases				
HIV infection				
Abdominal aortic aneurysm (one-time test)				

Source: Adapted from U.S. Preventive Services Task Force

As I said before, talk to your doctor about which of the above tests apply to you. He or she may suggest different testing depending upon your particular situation and medical history.

QUICK TAKEAWAYS: 5 STATS THAT CAN SAVE YOUR LIFE

(and your targets to shoot for)

1. Weight: BMI under 25, and waist of under 35 inches for women and under 40 inches for men.
2. Blood Pressure: At or below 120 over 80.
3. Cholesterol: get your total cholesterol under 200.
   - Get your LDL below 130 if you're at intermediate risk for heart disease.
   - Get your HDL above 50 if you're a woman and above 40 if you're a man.
   - And get your triglycerides to under 150.
4. Fasting Glucose: get under 100.
5. Calories: balance calories in and out with healthy eating and physical activity.

And don't forget: Absolute zero when it comes to smoking.

FIVE

MASTER THE MEDICAL PROCESS

I can think of nowhere on Earth I'd rather go to work than a hospital.

And if I were a patient I can think of nowhere else I'd rather not go than a hospital.

I am passionate about helping people get healthy. I cannot describe to you how rewarding and fulfilling it is to help save a fellow human being's life in the ER, to help heal a child's broken bone, or to help give a mother or father another forty years of life to enjoy with their family. There's no other feeling like it.

But let's face it, for most people, spending time in a hospital stinks. It is often a grueling experience when you're on the receiving end of the medical process. You're sick, weak, and uncomfortable. There are bells and buzzers going off all the time, carts banging in the hallway, and people poking and prodding you at all hours. And no matter how good your doctors and nurses are, you're usually confused, anxious, and incredibly eager or even desperate to get the heck out of there in one piece.

When I was growing up, I absolutely despised hospitals. My grandmother had a downward spiral in her health, entered a nursing home, and then was in and out of hospitals for the last years of her life. I visited her in the hospital and thought it was so scary—the sounds, sights, and smells combined to form a kind of nightmare to me as a child. I thought I would never want to work in one. I hated it.

I didn't have a very high opinion of doctors either. My pediatrician was a real old-school, cold-as-a-fish kind of guy. I'd march into his office and he'd barely say hello before commanding, "Turn to the left and cough."

The only time in my adult life when I was a patient in a hospital was when I was in college at Duke University, years before I became a doctor. I was cramming for final exams, neglected my health, and contracted a wicked form of pneumonia that knocked me flat on my butt. I spent three days in the infirmary with fever, sweats, and labored breathing. I lay in the hospital bed like a slug, knowing nothing of medicine, and I had no idea what questions to ask. I was a fairly intelligent guy but I had absolutely no clue what was going on. I kept my mouth shut.

"I'll let the doctors figure it out," I reasoned. "It's their job to fix me. I'm not going to pester them; I'll let them do their thing." I felt lucky that I was at Duke University, which is a great medical institution, and slowly I regained my strength. But let me tell you, I hated every minute of those three days.

Looking back on the experience, I can't believe how naïve and ignorant I was. I should have asked the doctors at least a dozen important questions. I should have asked them precisely what was going wrong with my body, how it got that way, what the alternative treatments and probable outcomes were. I should have paid attention to the medicines I was being given, and asked them how to prevent this from happening again.

I've been a doctor for a while now, and I've come to realize that it is the patient who has the real power in the doctor-patient relationship. You are the most crucial part of the medical process. This single insight has tremendous applications for your life: *Health and wellness isn't just what your doctor does when you go for a visit. It's everything you do in between.*

When it comes to fighting chronic disease, doctors don't really have that much power compared to patients. Doctors focus largely on treating illnesses once they've happened, but you have not only the power but the responsibility to stop illness and disease before it happens—by Being your own Health Guru, Eating to Savor Life, Treating Yourself to a Daily Vacation, and Nailing Your Health Stats. And that makes you about a million times more powerful and important than any doctor or scientist.

I've also come to realize that there are three simple ideas that will help you master the often frustrating and difficult process of interacting with the medical system. The three steps are: think like an ER doctor, make every moment of your doctor visit count, and ask the right questions so you enjoy the best possible hospital stay.

Step 1. *Think* like an ER doctor—stay out of the hospital!

The first step in mastering the medical process is to minimize the time you spend in the hospital or, better yet, stay out of it!

As an ER doctor I deal with the widest possible set of medical problems. But many of these situations will not happen to you if you follow the advice in this book and think like an ER doctor the way I do. It all boils down to being smart and reducing risks as much as possible.

In most aspects of my life, because of what I see in the emergency room, I take extra steps to protect myself against unnecessary risks and dangers. You should, too, and here's how:

Be a Healthy Germophobe. There are two ways of being a germophobe. You can be an obsessive-compulsive germo-fanatic like the famous Howard Hughes, sealed up in a dark room all your life in fear of deadly germs lurking everywhere, or wrapping your kids up in spacesuits before they venture out of the house. Not a good idea. The world is filled with bacteria, fungi, and germs—it's nature's plan.

But it's a great idea to be a healthy germophobe. That means taking strong, sensible precautions to avoid getting sick from harmful germs, such as those that cause a cold and the flu.

Doctors are famous for scrubbing up with soap and water, and you should absolutely make doing so a part of your healthy several-times-a-day routine. It sounds really mundane, but you've got to regularly wash your hands with soap and warm water for at least fifteen seconds, and avoid touching your eyes, nose, or mouth with your hands—that is the number one way to carry a harmful virus into your system.

If you shake someone's hand, remember that you now have whatever germs they have living on their hands on your hands, until you wash those germs off. You won't see me running off to wash my hands immediately after shaking everyone's hand, but you also won't see me rubbing my eyes or scratching my nose afterward either!

Travel presents another germ minefield. When I travel, I'm extra-careful of avoiding illness. I'll be sure to exercise on the road so I can keep my immune system in top shape and not overly vulnerable to getting sick, and I'm careful with the little things. For example, in my opinion, the dirtiest thing in a hotel room is the TV remote control. I doubt they ever bother to clean it. Everyone touches it, and germs can stay active and infectious on such a surface for many hours after the previous guest has left and you've checked in. You pick it up, and bang, you could catch a cold or the flu.

When you're traveling, especially overseas, you may become exposed to an amazing number of illnesses like malaria, dengue hemorrhagic fever, Japanese encephalitis, chikungunya fever, yellow fever, parasites, tick-borne diseases, and typhoid fever. Before traveling, ask your doctor what preventive shots or steps you should take, and check the Centers for Disease Control website (www .cdc.gov) for country-specific travelers' updates. You must be aware of these kinds of things. I'm not giving you this information to scare you, but so you're more conscious and can avoid untoward events.

Many sicknesses are caused by infection with bacteria or viruses, and you can stop them in their tracks by following these tips from me and from experts like the Joint Commission (formerly the Joint Commission on Accreditation of Healthcare Organizations) and the Centers for Disease Control:

TRAVIS L. STORK, M.D.

R̥ **DR. STORK'S TOP TIPS FOR BEING
A HEALTHY GERMOPHOBE**

- Realize that viral infections usually enter your body through your eyes, nose, and mouth. They are often transmitted by other people coughing or sneezing in your direction, or by your own hands picking up germs from infected people or surfaces.
- Avoid touching your eyes, nose, or mouth unless you've washed your hands.
- Try to avoid close contact with sick people who are coughing or sneezing.
- Cover your nose and mouth with a tissue when you cough or sneeze, and throw the tissue in the trash, or cough or sneeze into the crook of your elbow. Do not cough or sneeze onto your bare hands unless you can immediately wash them.
- Wash your hands thoroughly, and often, with soap and warm water for fifteen to twenty seconds. (I use good old-fashioned soap and try to avoid overusing antibacterial soap.) When soap and water are not available, alcohol-based disposable hand wipes or gel sanitizers may be used. I recommend using a sanitizer with at least 60 percent alcohol.

- Make sure doctors, dentists, and other health care providers clean their hands or wear gloves when treating you. They come into contact with lots of viruses and bacteria, so before they treat you, ask if they've cleaned their hands. They should wear clean gloves when they do things like take throat cultures, pull teeth, take blood, touch wounds or body fluids, and examine your mouth or private parts. Don't be afraid to ask them if they should be wearing gloves.
- Keep your immune system strong by getting plenty of physical activity, sleep, fluids, and following a healthy diet, especially when you're traveling.
- If you're sick with a flulike illness, the CDC recommends that you stay home for at least twenty-four hours after your fever is gone except to get medical care if needed or for other necessities. (Your fever should be gone without the use of a fever-reducing medicine.) Keep away from others as much as possible to keep from making others sick.
- When you're out and about or when you're traveling, if you've just washed your hands, try not to use your bare hands to touch commonly used and little-cleaned places. Examples include airplane bathroom door handles, elevator buttons, faucet and toilet handles, and doorknobs in general. You can't always do this gracefully and it isn't always easy to pull this off without looking like a contortionist or germo-fanatic, but wouldn't you rather stay healthy than look smooth? One simple trick: use the paper towel to turn off the faucet and open the bathroom door, and then throw it away.
- Check the Centers for Disease Control website www.cdc .gov for the latest advisories on infectious diseases, flu, and traveler's health.

- Get immunized—talk to your doctor about getting a seasonal flu vaccine shot, and don't forget to ask what other adult vaccinations you may need, such as tetanus and whooping cough.

Buckle up 100 percent of the time, and wear protective equipment. You'd think that in America we'd be past the point of having to remind people to buckle up, but millions of Americans still play games with their lives by ignoring this basic safety rule. I have witnessed horrific car, truck, motorcycle, and bicycle accidents, and I've seen the tragic price of carelessness and stupidity up close and personal.

A few years ago, the then-governor of New Jersey, Jon Corzine, a brilliant, wealthy investment banker-turned politician, got into his SUV and did what he usually did—he failed to wear his seat belt. When his SUV crashed, he was thrown around the inside of the vehicle like a rag doll. He was evacuated by helicopter to a Level 1 trauma center in critical condition with an open fracture of the left femur, eleven broken ribs, a broken sternum, a broken collarbone, a fractured lower vertebra, facial damage that required plastic surgery, and a breathing tube stuck down his throat. Many of these injuries could have been avoided if he'd just buckled up. He recovered, and went on to record a public service announcement where he said, "I'm New Jersey Governor Jon Corzine, and I should be dead."

On the flip side is a man I took care of who lost control of his motorcycle doing about 70 miles an hour in the fast lane. He flipped over and scraped along the pavement and the guardrail for 300 yards. Fortunately he was smart. Not only did he have his helmet on but he was wearing full-body protective gear from head to toe—wrist guards, pants, even neck protection. We patched him up in the ER and he walked out of the hospital a few hours later. Yes, he was extremely lucky, but he played a role in his own luck by being well prepared. You should, too.

Wise people don't just learn from their own mistakes—they learn from the mistakes of others. After what I've seen in the emergency room, I always wear my seat belt, and I insist everyone else in the car does, too. I'm on my bicycle a great deal, and I know that wearing a helmet can save lives. It infuriates me when I see parents allowing their kids to ride without a helmet. When I ski, you'd better believe I've always got a helmet on and I'm watching my speed. This wasn't always the case, but I've seen one too many lives tragically altered or cut short by head injuries. Is it worth it? No! Wear a helmet!

Never, ever use an electronic device while at the wheel of a moving vehicle. I would never dream of sending a text message when I'm behind the wheel of a moving vehicle. I acknowledge that I used to do this, but now I know better. I've seen the damage this can cause and, trust me, it's gruesome.

Tragically, many thousands of Americans are using their BlackBerries, iPhones, cell phones, and even computers while behind the wheel of their moving cars and trucks, which from a safety perspective is so dangerous as to stagger the imagination. The *New York Times* reported last year that "Studies show that someone who talks on the phone while driving is four times more likely to crash, even using a hands-free headset, than someone who is simply driving. The risks are even greater when sending text messages." The article went on to detail how crash victims are successfully suing the employers of such drivers for millions of dollars, and how the idea that you're more productive when electronically multitasking is a myth: "A growing body of research shows that splitting attention between activities like working and driving often leads to distracted conversations and bad decisions."

I believe we should have a 100 percent nationwide federal ban on all texting, phoning, emailing, computer work, or similar activity from behind the wheel of a moving vehicle—no exceptions, no excuses.

In the meantime, you should enforce the ban on yourself and your family. The point isn't to go through life in a state of paralytic fear, but to be careful and avoid unnecessary and flagrantly life-threatening risks. The reality is this: patients usually say the same thing to me after an accident—"It happened so fast." In the split second it takes to look down at your phone . . . wham! It's too late.

Tackle emergencies before they happen—be prepared. People rarely think about emergencies until they happen. It's not in our nature to automatically plan for disasters before they strike. But you should always be prepared, so that if something bad does happen, you're as protected as you can be—and you spend as little time in doctors' offices and hospitals as possible.

Let me tell you an ER doctor's secret. One of the first things we'll do if you're rushed into the ER and you're unconscious is we will rifle through your pockets, wallet, or purse. I'm urgently looking for your key medical information—a few basic bits of info that will help me give you better care and maybe save your life. Sometimes I find it. But most of the time I don't. People usually don't think to carry this information with them, and that omission can burn up critical time in the ER while the staff has to start piecing the information together from scratch.

Take a few minutes to create what I call your "Instant Portable Medical Chart," or "Everything They Need to Know About You (or Your Child) in an Emergency—in 30 Seconds or Less." This way, if trouble happens, you or the medical personnel won't be fumbling around and wasting precious time, and you'll get the best possible medical care. Here's what to include:

Travis L. Stork, M.D.

R   **Dr. Stork's Portable Medical Chart**

(aka, the One List You Should

Always Have on You)

Write or type this information on a piece of paper or an index card, fold it up, and stick it in your purse or wallet. (You can also ask your primary care doctor's office to give you all the information for this list at your next doctor visit.) When seconds count, these six pieces of information can save your life.

- Capsule summary of your medical conditions, including previous surgeries.
- List of prescription medications and any other pills you take, with dosages—including vitamins, herbs, aspirin, and over-the-counter (OTC) drugs.
- List of any allergies to medications you have.
- If you smoke or drink, and how much on the average day.
- Capsule family history—your mother and father's medical conditions, and if deceased, their age at death and cause of death as well as any other important and pertinent family history.
- Phone numbers for your emergency contacts—your doctor, your family.

Kid's Backpack Version

Write or type this information on a piece of paper or an index card, fold it up, and stick it in your child's schoolbag or coat pocket.

- Capsule summary of any medical conditions, including previous surgeries.

- List of prescription medications and any other pills, with dosages—including vitamins, herbs, aspirin, and OTC drugs.
- List of any allergies to medications.
- Phone numbers for emergency contacts.

Some day in the not-too-distant future, hopefully, we will all have standardized microchips, wristbands, or web tools that will instantly link our medical information to any doctor or hospital that needs it. There are already some fascinating new ventures to help you collect your personal medical records and information in one easy-to-access place online, like these services you might want to try out:

Microsoft Health Vault: http://healthvault.com

Google Health: www.google.com/health

WebMD Personal Health Record: www.webmd.com/phr

Establish a home base for your medical care. Many people don't realize something very important when it comes to mastering the medical process: to optimize the quality of your health care, you should try to consolidate it as much as possible at a single institution. In other words, your primary care doctor should ideally have an affiliation with a leading medical facility, and whenever feasible, that's where you want to consider going first for scheduled surgeries and tests, as well as for emergencies.

People don't realize that, by and large, most medical institutions are not yet hooked up with each other instantly and electronically when it comes to patients' medical records. They're usually hooked up inside their own facility, but not across different ones. That may make no sense in our hyperlinked day and age, but it's an unfortunate fact of our much-stressed medical system.

For example, if your doctor was affiliated with Vanderbilt University Medical Center and you came into our ER, I would instantly be able to call up all your medical information on the computer—your surgeries, allergies, medications, whether or not you smoke, if you're married, etc. This is an excellent scenario for both doctor and patient.

But let's say you "institution hop" or "institution shop," and you come into the Vanderbilt ER for the first time with several health complaints because you heard great things about the facility. However, since all your records are over at another hospital, you're not doing yourself any favors, because I'm going to have to spend precious time reconstructing all your crucial information. I see this happen all the time.

Recently I saw someone in the Vanderbilt ER who walked in and complained of a pain in his abdomen. A week earlier he'd had a surgery performed at a different hospital and now he was having a postsurgical complication. He wasn't even sure what the surgery was called. I couldn't reach his surgeon easily because it was after hours and nobody was answering in the medical records department of the hospital he had been at the previous week. We were able to help him, but only after slowly and painstakingly piecing together his medical history.

The lesson: think ahead, and have a plan. The plan can be as simple as finding a primary care doctor you like and trust, asking them what institution they're affiliated with and if they share computerized electronic medical records. In this way, you can determine if your medical records will be available to all of your health care providers, whether you are going to your primary doctor, to the ER, or to see a specialist. Hopefully they will be.

ASK DR. STORK

Question: How can I best prepare for an emergency?

Answer: I have three tips for you: locate an AED, learn CPR, and pack two emergency kits.

An AED is an automatic external defibrillator. It is a relatively new, and increasingly widespread, portable, "idiot-proof" computerized machine that can save the life of someone who is suffering sudden cardiac arrest (SCA). These are fantastic devices that in an emergency any adult can open up and use, because the machine instructs you how to use it. (They are best used by someone who is trained, but prior use is not necessary.)

Every day in America, some 1,000 people experience SCA, and because time is so short, 95 percent of victims die before medical help can get to them. An AED can help sharply increase odds of survival. The machine diagnoses a person's heart rhythm, checks if the rhythm needs a shock, and, if necessary, delivers a lifesaving electrical current to get the rhythm back to normal. It uses text and voice prompts with instructions to tell the rescuer the steps to take. Many places like office buildings, airports, sports arenas, and shopping malls are now equipped with AEDs.

One of my best friends is an ER doctor. He was working out in the gym one day and saw a guy lifting weights who suddenly collapsed. Being an ER doctor, he obviously knew what to do, but he didn't know where the AED was located. Luckily, the staff at the health club knew exactly where the AED was in their building and retrieved it immediately. My friend performed CPR until it arrived and then used it to shock the heart back to a normal rhythm. Days later the gentleman walked out of the hospital no worse for wear, having suffered what would have been a fatal heart attack if not for the AED.

Take a minute and ask the staff at your health club, workplace, or any other location that you frequent where the AED is. The faster you can locate the AED, the faster you can provide help to someone in a crisis.

The second tip is to learn CPR, which could help you save the life of someone in your family or a perfect stranger. The sooner you administer effective CPR before defibrillation in an emergency, the better. A victim's odds of surviving drop 7 percent to 10 percent with each minute that passes without CPR and defibrillation. According to the American Heart Association, few people are revived after the ten minute mark.

Both the American Heart Association (1-877-AHA-4CPR) and the American Red Cross (www.redcross.org) have training courses in both CPR and in using an AED. You should spend an afternoon taking the training—it is a very wise investment of your time.

Finally, I suggest that you either buy or assemble two emergency kits to have on hand—a safety kit and a first aid kit. The American Red Cross has put together excellent tips for putting together the potentially lifesaving kits, tips available at www.redcross.org.

The Bottom Line: Locate the nearest AED, take a CPR course, and build an emergency kit and a first aid kit.

Step 2: Make every moment of your doctor visit count.

Imagine this scenario: You've noticed something wrong with your health and you've made an appointment with your doctor. You're in the exam room, the doctor has finally arrived, and you've got his or her attention for the next few precious minutes—that's about it.

You know you must communicate your situation clearly to the doctor, but suddenly you get flummoxed.

You've been anticipating this visit for days, yet somehow, the sight of a doctor with a stethoscope around his or her neck paralyzes your thought process. You can't remember key details. It seems like the doctor is talking in a foreign language and you can't pick up a word that's being said. You forget a key piece of your family history, and you're afraid that when you're in the car on the way home a half hour from now, you'll have five critical questions you forgot to ask.

If the doctor is good, he or she will make you feel relaxed and bring you back on track, however, there may still not be enough time to address all of your concerns. The American health care system is so broken that many doctors are overwhelmed by the volume of patients they must see and the paperwork they have to fill out. The result is precious little meaningful time with patients. This is not your doctor's fault—we all wish we had more time with our patients. Personally I wish I had time to persuade many of my patients to take better care of themselves once I've stabilized their condition or fixed their health crisis, but suddenly I hear on the intercom, "Doctor Stork, we need you in Trauma Bay Three. Gunshot wound to the head," and I've got to run.

So how can you possibly get good health care when you may only have five productive minutes with your doctor? The key is to understand that your doctor is not in charge of your health care. You are.

I have seen thousands of patients over the years, and in the process I've noticed a surprising and extremely important component to getting the best care: you need to realize that it's your responsibility as a patient to tell your doctor a clear, concise, and accurate story. We doctors call this story "the history."

It sounds amazingly simple, doesn't it?

Unfortunately, a great many people come in and have difficulty providing a good history of what's going on. Obviously, there are extenuating circumstances in which providing a history is impossible (i.e., the patient is in extreme distress or unconscious); however, by providing a good history, you can sharply improve the quality of your care.

The reality is you could send five different doctors in to see a patient and the docs might come out with five different stories. One doctor will say, "I think it's a fever of unknown origin." Another will say, "You know what? They've had a pain up their leg for two weeks." Yet another will note, "There's a severe headache with vomiting." The next doctor may say, "The patient is feeling really depressed." I've actually seen this happen many times.

What's a "bad story" to tell your doctor? It's a story that is too vague or misses important details, with too much time spent on extraneous information. I once had a patient in the ER tell me a bad story that went something like this:

> "Dr. Stork, four weeks ago, when I was picking my husband up from the store, I noticed that we were low on gas. I took the car to the gas station, where I noticed the car's windows were dirty. So I filled up the gas and went through the car wash. As the car was being cleaned, I noticed this little pain in the back of my leg. So I drove home and made a few cocktails. They were really delicious, and my husband and I wound up having a nice dinner. After dessert we went to a movie and, oh, my leg wasn't really hurting me any more at that point, but then the next day when I woke up, I noticed something. I went to Starbucks— normally I get black coffee but this day I decided to get a hot tea—then afterward, when I was walking home, I noticed the pain came back. And then . . ."

I couldn't have been more confused! The right way to tell the story would have been:

> "Four weeks ago, I had a pain in the back of my right leg in the calf area. I don't remember hurting it. It lasted for maybe eight hours but slowly went away. I was fine until three days

ago, when the pain came back, only stronger, and it went up to the back of my knee. It especially hurts when I press on it. Over the past twenty-four hours it has gotten slightly red and even a little swollen."

That's a great story. The patient outlined the problem clearly and concisely, so her doctor has plenty of time to dig deeper.

Doctors often interrupt their patients within the first ten seconds of an appointment. That is not a good thing, but if you go to the doctor's office prepared, it shouldn't happen. If you come to see me with symptoms of chest pain, something that might kill you, it's really not a good time to tell me about the hemorrhoids you had a year ago while on vacation in Costa Rica!

Similarly, you don't want to show up with no information other than "my chest hurts." I don't want to interrupt you while you're telling your story, but if you aren't telling a good story, I have to jump in, in order to get your treatment started. Instead, the right way to tell your doctor about the problem is to be specific, like this: "It started last night. There were three episodes of chest pain lasting ten minutes each. It's a sharp pain, and it's worse when I take a deep breath." Excellent story! The story demonstrates that the patient has already thought through exactly what's going on, and maybe asked their spouse to take notes so they can get the points across clearly in the doctor's office or the ER. Now I can get straight to work getting you healthy.

Let's say you're taking your sick child to the pediatrician. A bad story is: "Doctor, my kid is just not acting normal. I don't know how many days it's been, but I think it's been going on for a while." I'll ask how many days the child has seemed to be behaving strangely, and the response is: "I don't know; it's definitely been a while, though."

A better story would be: "A few days ago he didn't seem to be eating well. I didn't think much of it, but then last night he had a fever of one hundred two degrees and he started vomiting. Since that time he hasn't wanted to play. I gave him some Tylenol but he threw it up and doesn't want to eat or drink, and other than that I don't know what's going on. Oh, and he developed a rash on his cheeks last night." Perfect! Now I have a clear background story. I can ask follow-up questions and figure out what's going on in a timely way.

Do your homework before going to the doctor. Bring along a list of your medicines and your allergies. Write down on a piece of paper a few short sentences describing the history of your symptoms, and the top three to five most important questions you want to ask. Some people overresearch their health issues on the web and come in with a list of twenty or more questions—that's not a good use of your time, as it increases the risk that this crucial conversation with your doctor will veer off course.

The patients who get the best care are the ones who are invested in their own care and have a good, honest relationship with their doctors. Never be embarrassed to tell your doctor anything—believe me, we've heard it all before! Be completely open and tell your doctor of any concerns you have. You should not exaggerate or try to be overly stoic. If your doctor is talking about your blood pressure being a little high but he or she forgets to ask about how stressful your life is, guess what? You should bring it up. If you don't have an open and truthful relationship with your doctor, it may be time to find a new one. And like most relationships, the key to success is communicating effectively.

Now here's an idea that may seem completely out of left field, but I absolutely believe it can help you get better medical care: think of your doctor as your employee or contractor, which in a sense he or she actually is, and be both a boss and a leader to them.

You should inspire your doctor.

What do great leaders do? They inspire people to do great things. I believe you can do the same thing with your doctor. Doctors are first and foremost human beings, with all the human flaws, weaknesses, and sensitivities. They can get impressed, excited, motivated, and joyful when, in partnership with the patient, they help a patient get better. That's why most doctors go into medicine in the first place— they like nothing more than helping people get healthy.

But believe me, there's nothing more frustrating for a doctor than a patient who doesn't follow through. Many times doctors can feel like they're fighting a losing battle.

For example, let's say during a visit I ask a patient to stop smoking, or to improve their eating habits, or to exercise or take a certain medicine. If I see them again in six months and they've ignored all of my advice, I sometimes feel helpless, dejected, and even crushed. I'll wonder if I care more about my patient's health than they do. I can offer advice and motivation, but the follow-through is completely dependent on the patient.

It's your job as a patient to take charge of your own wellness, to get very serious about eating right and exercising, to work to nail your health stats, and to master the medical process. It's your job to inspire your doctor to make them excited to give you the best care possible. It may sound ridiculous, but that really is your responsibility as a patient. I'm a doctor and a patient, and I know it's my job when I'm on the receiving end of treatment to be the best possible patient for my doctors. Again, doctors are human and we get excited to see patients who are invested in the process. If you master your own health and conquer preventable sickness before it happens, your doctor will truly feel like they're your partner in building your healthy future. We'll always do our best for you and inspire you to make better choices, but there's nothing quite like the feeling of taking care of a patient who is an active part of the process.

Step 3: Ask the right questions ahead of time, so you have the best possible hospital stay and medical care.

No matter how well you take care of yourself, there may be times when you have no choice but to spend time in the hospital. Emergencies and unexpected illnesses can and do occur, and often they require surgery or major treatment in a hospital setting.

In the United States we have some of the best doctors and nurses in the world. But everyone knows the health care system is far from perfect and mistakes can and do happen. As the CEO of your own medical care, you should be the boss and ask the right questions ahead of time, to reduce the chance of errors occurring and to get the best possible care when you're in the hospital. It's a simple fact: studies show that patients who are more involved with their care tend to have better outcomes.

The keys are to ask questions, speak up, and be the boss of your own care.

The following are checklists of my tips and tips from experts like the Agency for Healthcare Research and Quality on how to master each step of the medical process, including your hospital stay, should you need one:

HOW TO GET THE MOST OUT OF YOUR INTERACTIONS WITH A DOCTOR

- Write down your questions beforehand. List the most important ones first to make sure they get asked and answered.
- Give information; don't wait to be asked! Tell your doctor what you think he or she needs to know.
- Tell your doctor your personal information—even if it makes you feel embarrassed or uncomfortable. Include your personal and family health histories, your diet and exercise habits, your

sexual practices if relevant to the discussion, and if you use tobacco, alcohol, or other drugs.

- Always bring any medicines you are taking, or a list of those medicines (include when and how often you take them) and what strength. Talk about any allergies or reactions you have had to medicines.
- Tell your doctor about any herbal products, vitamins, or over-the-counter drugs you use, as well as alternative medicines or treatments you receive.
- Bring other medical information, such as X-ray films, test results, and medical records if you are coming from a different hospital or practice.
- Ask questions. If you don't, your doctor will assume you understand everything that was said.
- Don't be afraid to interrupt your doctor to clarify a point, and don't be afraid to ask them to explain it again "in plain English." Ask your doctor to draw pictures if that might help to explain something.
- Consider bringing a friend or family member to help you understand and/or remember instructions.
- Take notes. Some doctors don't mind if you bring a tape recorder to help you remember things, but always ask first.
- When your doctor writes you a prescription, make sure you can read it. If you can't read your doctor's handwriting, your pharmacist might not be able to either.
- Ask for written instructions for your treatment, including medications.
- Ask for a copy of your medical records for your home file.
- Once you leave the doctor's office, it's up to you to follow up by doing the following:
  - If you have questions, call.

- If your symptoms get worse, or if you have problems with your medicine, call.
- If you had tests and do not hear from your doctor, call for your test results.
- If your doctor said you need to have certain tests, make appointments at the lab or other offices to get them done promptly.
- If your doctor said you should see a specialist, then do it.

Potential Questions for Your Doctor

When your doctor gives you a diagnosis:

What is my diagnosis?

_____

What is the technical name of my disease or condition, and what does it mean in plain English?

_____

What is my prognosis (outlook for the future)?

_____

What changes will I need to make?

_____

Is there a chance that someone else in my family might get the same condition?

_____

Will I need special help at home for my condition?

_____

Is there any treatment?

_____

What are my treatment options?

_____

How soon do I need to make a decision about treatment?

_____

What are the benefits and risks associated with my treatment options?

_____

Is there a clinical trial (research study) that is right for me?

_____

Will I need any additional tests?

_____

What organizations and resources do you recommend for support and information?

_____

When your doctor recommends treatment:

What are my treatment options?

_____

What do you recommend?

_____

Is the treatment painful?

_____

How can the pain be controlled?

_____

What are the benefits and risks of this treatment?

_____

How much does this treatment cost?

_____

Will my health insurance cover the treatment?

_____

What are the expected results?

_____

When should I see results from the treatment?

_____

What are the chances the treatment will work?

_____

Are there any side effects?

_____

What can be done about them?

_____

How soon do I need to make a decision about treatment?

_____

What happens if I choose to have no treatment at all?

_____

Before you enter the hospital for surgery:

Why do I need surgery?

_____

What kind of surgery do I need?

_____

What will you be doing?

_____

What are the benefits and risks of having this surgery?

_____

Have you done this surgery before?

_____

How successful is this surgery?

_____

Which hospital is best for this surgery?

_____

Will the surgery hurt?

_____

Will I need anesthesia?

_____

How long will the surgery take?

_____

Do you follow a surgical safety checklist?

_____

Will there by physical aftereffects from the surgery?

_____

How long will it take me to recover?

_____

How long will I be in the hospital?

_____

What will happen after the surgery?

_____

How much will the surgery cost?

_____

Will my health insurance cover the surgery?

_____

Is there some other way to treat my condition?

_____

What will happen if I wait or don't have this surgery?

_____

Is there any alternative to the surgery?

_____

Where can I get a second opinion?

_____

Tips for Once You're in the Hospital

- Ask for, and read, a copy of the American Hospital Association's *A Patient's Bill of Rights.*
- If possible, bring along a family member or buddy to help you through the process, help be an advocate, and act as your "eyes and ears."

- Ask if the hospital has a patient advocate on staff, and if they can stop by to introduce themselves before your procedure so you know who they are and how to reach them.
- Ask every member of the hospital staff who comes into your room to introduce themselves and describe their role in your care, so you understand how your hospital team works.
- Ask every doctor, nurse, and visitor who comes into your room to wash their hands. That's the #1 way to stop the spread of infections.
- Make sure that the hospital staff consults your wristbands before administering treatment or meds, they contain your ID and details on your care.
- Review major details of your operation—including the site of the surgery—with the surgeon before it happens, to minimize the chances of a mistake.
- If you think something is wrong, speak up.
- Be sure you clearly understand your discharge instructions and details regarding your medications. Ask for written instructions from your doctor or the medical staff and make sure you understand them fully.

Mastering the Medical Process: Quick and Easy Takeaways

Here are the basics to remember so you'll stay out of the ER!

1. Think like an ER doctor: prevent problems before they happen, and get the checkups and tests you need, so you spend as little time in the medical system as possible.

2. Make every moment of your doctor visit count: tell the right story and inspire your doctor.

3. Ask the right questions ahead of time, so you have the best possible hospital stay and receive the best medical care.

OPEN YOUR MIND TO ALTERNATIVES

I am a huge believer in alternative approaches to wellness. Proven alternatives, that is.

In fact, I believe if people fully tapped the power of the two most incredibly powerful alternative medicines available on Planet Earth—healthy eating and regular physical activity—half the pharmaceutical companies would have to shut their doors. And that would be a good thing. Why? Because most of us would be living much happier lives, and spending much less time trapped in the hospital by disease and disability.

My personal philosophy regarding alternative medicine is extremely simple, and I suggest you consider adopting it yourself:

Dr. Stork's 3 Key Ideas Regarding Alternative Medicine

- Be simultaneously open-minded and ruthlessly skeptical.

- Demand of alternative medicine the same quality of information that you should demand of conventional medicine. Anecdotes, testimonials, and sales talk don't count—you cannot play guessing games with your health.

- Demand the best research and most qualified expert opinions on alternative medicines, and ask the toughest possible questions.

I try to take charge of my own health by using any effective "alternatives" I can find. I like to stay out of the medical system as a patient, so I exercise regularly and I eat really healthy the majority of the time. I take a multivitamin and a fish oil supplement every day (more on this later in the chapter). I "detox" my home by using as few harsh chemicals as possible. I practice deep breathing, which is a form of meditation, when I get stressed out, and I am a big supporter of yoga, Pilates, and any other form of movement and relaxation that we know improves our physiology and may effectively reduce our need for pharmaceutical intervention. There are thousands of other alternative approaches to wellness, and it is always interesting to evaluate them. When I'm considering something new, I look at the evidence, and if I think something is risky or a waste of money, I'll say so.

My mind is wide open to new approaches, to ancient wisdom, and to both critics and supporters of the current medical establishment. I believe so-called Western medicine has traditionally been too closed-minded. Medical doctors are sometimes guilty of not even considering a nonmedical approach to a disease or illness, although this is slowly changing. For the record, complementary medicine is technically defined as being used together with conventional medicine, while alternative medicine is used in place of it, but for purposes of this chapter, I am referring to alternative medicine as anything that is unconventional, whether it is used with conventional medicine or not.

I am incredibly proud of doctors in America. I believe they are the best in the world. Foreign medical grads desperately want to train in America because our training is second to none! Doctors here do amazing work and are devoted to giving their patients the best possible care. One of the things I am most proud of about *The Doctors* is that we get to bring doctors on the program from each and every medical specialty, to show the world a side of doctors many don't always see: the compassion that drives patient care, medical research, and innovation.

But let's face it, doctors are human. Doctors can be wrong and they can make mistakes. Sometimes doctors don't communicate well or empathize well with patients. Some can be closed-minded and even arrogant. They can be too prone to automatically dispensing medication rather than looking for the deeper causes and roots of illnesses. On top of this, pharmaceutical companies can make mistakes by releasing drugs that turn out to be dangerous and then have to be withdrawn. And, while hopefully only in rare instances, some pharmaceutical companies have reportedly interfered with or even ghostwritten research to skew the results to sell more medication or certain procedures.

The fact is, no matter how brilliant and heroic the doctor is, or how effective the medication or surgery may be, sometimes modern medicine just plain doesn't work. For example, new research indicates that even some standard procedures like angioplasty and coronary bypass surgery turn out to not have quite the effect on prolonging life that we thought.

Experts disagree all the time, and medical wisdom is very much a moving target that changes over time as new knowledge is gained. Some of the standard wisdom I learned in medical school has now been completely debunked. I am truly amazed by how much we know in medicine, but sometimes I'm more amazed at how little we know. Now is an exciting time to be in medicine, because we are finally starting to uncover some medical truths we never quite understood. And one of those truths may very well be that the simple things can sometimes make the biggest difference. Consider this: the way we performed CPR for many years now looks like it may be fairly ineffective. New studies suggest there may be a benefit to performing only chest compressions in the field, without giving rescue breaths. This is such a drastic change from conventional teaching and wisdom that it makes you wonder what to believe anymore.

For all these reasons, many of us look for alternative ideas to complement or even replace traditional medicine. The term "complementary and alternative medicine," or CAM, has come to encompass a gigantic grab bag of theories, including good and bad ideas, from transformative breakthroughs to completely bogus quackery. CAM is an over $30 billion industry, and almost 40 percent of adult Americans are using at least one alternative concept or therapy, like taking vitamins or herbal supplements, doing yoga or meditation, or using acupuncture.

Some CAM ideas are brilliant and have the power to revolutionize your health in a positive direction. Other CAM ideas are downright dangerous and have the potential to injure or even kill you. A well-known example of this is the supplement ephedra, a traditional Chinese herbal remedy once widely sold in health food stores that was banned by the Food and Drug Administration in 2004 after being linked to a number of fatalities, including the death of Baltimore Orioles pitcher Steve Belcher.

I am almost embarrassed to admit this, but I used to take ephedra in medical school after a long, sleep-deprived night on call. As you've probably heard, the hours can be really brutal in the hospital. I'd be so tired after being up for thirty-six hours, that the supercharged, caffeinelike effects of ephedra would allow me stay awake for a few more hours despite major sleep deprivation. So I'd take some ephedra as I was leaving the hospital. This gave me just enough energy to go exercise and enjoy a few hours of the evening before passing out from exhaustion. At the time, the herb was not well studied and I thought it was the best thing since sliced bread. It helped me enjoy a terrific workout after being awake for a day and a half. Little did I know I was putting my life at risk!

This was an over-the-counter supplement that I bought at the grocery store as easily as a pack of chewing gum, and it had the power to inflict severe liver damage or even death on me. The lesson I learned: some supplements can be more dangerous than prescription medicines because they are largely unregulated.

If that doesn't scare you, it should! I am no longer naïve and you shouldn't be either.

The problem with much of alternative medicine is that in many cases, there is little scientific evidence that it works, or that it is safe. There are several reasons for this. One is that an alternative simply hasn't been researched properly. A lot of research is driven by the almighty dollar, so sometimes alternative approaches take a little longer to get "researched." Acupuncture is a great example of an alternative treatment about which many in the medical community were dubious, until research ultimately suggested it can be effective in certain conditions. I admit that just because a substance or treatment hasn't been scientifically tested yet doesn't mean it doesn't work. However, as was the case with ephedra, it does mean it could be dangerous and you may very well be putting your life at risk (not to mention wasting your money).

Also, in my opinion many alternative treatments simply don't work. And the companies selling the alternative treatment know a good randomized, controlled trial may just put them out of business. In that case, they often won't put forth the resources necessary to get a study done. Instead, it's much easier to market the alternative product colorfully with a label that might read like this:

A special herb from the rain forests of the Amazon with a natural, organic ability to erase your wrinkles, lower your stress, increase your vitality, improve blood flow, boost your metabolism, burn off fat, melt away the pounds, decrease waist size, strengthen your muscles, and boost your libido.

Excuse me—says who? Is there a shred of good evidence to support any of that?

We consumers can be really enthusiastic and trusting people, and with a sweet-as-molasses sales pitch like the above on labels, however bogus it may be, it's easy to see why consumers waste so much money on unproven and potentially dangerous treatments. And why would a business ever want to commission a study to back their claims (probably false) if they are already making money hand over fist selling it?

But in America we love stories, and a great story can sound a lot more compelling than actual good evidence. If we see a powerful infomercial or hear a seductive sales pitch or a rave testimonial review from our brother-in-law for an alternative medical approach, we can be persuaded. Or we can convince ourselves that there's a secret conspiracy between big pharmaceutical companies and the medical establishment to suppress an alternative remedy. That's a sexy idea, but I don't think it happens very often.

Here is the paradox: despite the lack of evidence to back up many alternative treatments and therapies, or even good scientific theories to support them, for millions of Americans they do often seem to work. In many cases, however, the alternative's apparent effectiveness may not be the result of any healing power, but from one or more of a number of what I'll call "phantom" reasons that were identified by brain-behavior expert Barry Beyerstein, PhD, in a fascinating paper in the March 2001 edition of *Academic Medicine* titled "Alternative Medicine and Common Errors of Reasoning," which I outline here:

- The illness can be a cyclic condition in which symptoms have a natural upturn of improvement. For example, arthritis, multiple sclerosis, asthma, allergies, migraines, and many dermatologic, gynecologic, and gastrointestinal complaints normally have ups and downs, and a bogus alternative remedy can be misinterpreted as the reason for an upturn. (This is similar to how so many people claim antibiotics or herbal remedies help their colds go away when in reality, the natural course of a cold is to go away on its own after a few days, so you would get better regardless. But people who take an antibiotic or herbal remedy tend to credit the pill, even though it had absolutely nothing to do with them getting over their cold.)

- The placebo effect of a patient's belief in an alternative remedy can psychologically reduce pain by redirecting attention, increasing feelings of control and positive expectations, and easing anxiety, even if the alternative treatment being used is biologically useless.

- The charismatic, kind, and enthusiastic personalities that many alternative healers have can give the patient a mental uplift, enhance the placebo effect, reduce stress, encourage the patient to improve their lifestyle habits, and speed natural recovery, which is not a specific effect of the alternative therapy itself.

Many supporters of CAM argue that because conventional medicine is often imperfect, or influenced by pharmaceutical companies, or flat out wrong, alternatives should be considered equally valid or even preferred. But as Professor Beyerstein argued, "this criticism does nothing to enhance the credibility of CAM, for merely arguing that they're as bad as we are offers no positive evidence in favor of one's own pet belief." Plus, he added, there's a huge institutional difference between the two worlds: "Unlike the alternatives, scientific medicine is institutionally committed to weeding out treatments that fail to pass muster, and it does not cling to procedures and theories contradicted by the basic sciences."

I'm in favor of any alternative approach that works for someone, as long as it's not a rip-off, has no major known side effects, and has some basis in good medical evidence or scientific theory. I believe in evidence-based medicine, not faith-only-based medicine. If an alternative seems to be working, like acupuncture, let's test it and see if it passes. If it shows promise, like acupuncture does for low back pain, let's use it in those conditions where it seems helpful.

Too often doctors get used to doing things a certain way and we don't always accept the idea that other ways can work. You don't want a doctor who is automatically dismissive of all alternatives without looking at the evidence or theories behind it. But, if your doctor is skeptical about an alternative medical idea, that's a good thing. You want a doctor who has an open mind and listens to alternatives, but you also want that doctor to have a healthy, productive skepticism toward any alternative medical approach, as well as any unproven conventional approach. You should want to hear all the pros and cons. Then the two of you can talk it through and figure out what the best treatment path is for you. Healthy skepticism is the basis of good medicine and good decision-making. If your doctor has a basis for feeling that a certain alternative is unproven, or a rip-off, or medically dangerous, you want them to tell you that. They're doing you a favor!

If you're in my ER and you tell me about an alternative medical treatment that I can't find good data for, well, I don't want to burst your bubble, but I'll absolutely tell you what I think the medical reality is. I don't know everything and I'm learning new things every day—no doctor knows everything—but I won't flatter you by blowing smoke up your nose and telling you what you want to hear.

Sometimes patients misconstrue a doctor's healthy skepticism for irrational closed-mindedness, and they look to other sources for answers. For example, every day thousands of Americans flock into health food stores and ask for medical advice. Okay, I stop into health food stores all the time to pick up an energy bar or a snack, but a health food store can be a dangerous place to get medical advice.

It is not uncommon for people to ask the health food sales staff questions like, "What do you have for headaches?" "What can I buy that will give me more energy?" "I've got pain in my joints from weightlifting. Which of these herbal bone health formulas works the best?" "How much weight can I lose with this detox cleansing product?"

The unfortunate truth is that health food stores can be a wilderness of misinformation often populated by people who are regurgitating sales pitches to you that come from health product manufacturers. It might be fun to listen to marketing pitches, but if I were you I would never buy an alternative remedy without checking out the facts first.

I'm going to get on my high horse for a minute.

I hate to say this, but there are some people who claim to practice alternative medicine and who are hacks, quacks, and frauds. They make up some bogus credential, hang out a sign, and start charging fees for giving health advice. Unfortunately, it's legal. Here's the big problem: these people will tell you exactly what you want to hear. They'll talk your ear off about how amazing their services and supplements are and how "this new treatment is only eighty dollars a month but it's changing all of my clients' lives."

Please spare me the miracle product sales pitch and just give me the facts!

Celebrities are another source of alternative medical advice, some of which is great and some of which is bogus. Most celebrities have zero medical training, and they should never be your main source of health advice. As your own health guru, armed with the right information, you are potentially a thousand times smarter on the subject of health than they are.

Your main source of medical advice should be an open-minded medical doctor, period. If your doc isn't open-minded, find a new one who is. They're out there.

In the pages that follow I'll take you on a high-speed tour of some of the highlights of the world of complementary and alternative medicine. I'll touch on the alternatives that, in my opinion, you should stay away from; those you should check out; and tips for evaluating alternative treatments in your own life, which you should always do in conjunction with your doctor.

Alternative: Vitamin Supplements

I have rather shocking news for you. Vitamins are a $10 billion-plus industry, and there are thousands upon thousands of vitamin supplements on the market today, but the large majority of them have not been proven to be effective. While research and opinions change over time, the best, latest research indicates that most people probably don't need extra vitamins in supplement form, especially if you eat a healthy overall diet. With some possible exceptions (listed on page 194), you shouldn't bleed your bank account on vitamin supplements.

For many years, a lot of alternative medicine figures, as well as mainstream health experts, assumed that antioxidant supplements like vitamins A, C, and E worked to reduce the risks of chronic disease. The assumption was based on the theory that antioxidant vitamins scavenged or mopped up free radicals, chemicals in our bodies linked to disease and aging. But it turns out that it may not be that simple.

The newest, best research suggests that taking vitamin supplements like A, C, E and beta-carotene does not help your body fight cancer, cardiovascular disease, or chronic disease. Similarly, for many years, megadoses of vitamin C were thought to fight colds, but this idea has been thoroughly disproven. In some cases vitamin supplements may even be harmful to our health. In 2004, for example, the American Heart Association warned that taking 400 International Units (IU) a day or more of vitamin E could increase the risk of death.

The negative research on certain vitamin supplements has been fairly relentless in recent years. In 2006, a major conference held by the National Institutes of Health reviewed all the evidence and concluded in the *Annals of Internal Medicine* that "evidence is insufficient to prove the presence or absence of benefits from use of multivitamin and mineral supplements to prevent cancer and chronic disease." The evidence also suggested that multivitamin and mineral supplementation has no significant effect in the primary prevention of hypertension, cardiovascular disease, and cataracts.

In 2008, an analysis by the prestigious Cochrane Collaboration asked the questions "Can antioxidants prevent disease in healthy people? Can they prevent recurrences in people with cancer, heart disease, or other illnesses?" The results, which were based on gold-standard randomized trials involving hundreds of thousands of people, was that the researchers found "no evidence to support antioxidant supplements for primary or secondary prevention. Vitamin A, beta-carotene, and vitamin E may increase mortality." Data published in the February 9, 2009 *Archives of Internal Medicine* from the Women's Health Initiative trial, which tracked multivitamin use among over 161,000 postmenopausal women, found no benefit from multivitamin supplements against cancer, cardiovascular disease, or overall mortality.

And, also in 2009, the National Cancer Institute had to stop a major study of selenium and vitamin E's potential effects against prostate cancer (the Selenium and Vitamin E Cancer Prevention Trial, or SELECT), a study involving over 35,000 men, when no beneficial effects were seen. The Institute also had to prematurely stop another large-scale trial when beta-carotene supplements were linked to a higher incidence of lung cancer and mortality in those at risk through asbestos exposure or smoking.

My Opinion: In general, you should get your nutrients from food, not pills. The majority of vitamin supplements have no proven benefits.

Healthy eating patterns based on whole foods like veggies, fruit, legumes, and whole grains give your body a fantastically complex symphony of health-promoting, disease-fighting vitamins, minerals, phytochemicals, and fiber, a symphony that is much more powerful than any vitamin taken as a pill.

There are always exceptions. Some supplements may have benefits for some people. Here are some examples you should talk to your doctor about, according to experts such as the American Institute for Cancer Research, the American Heart Association, and the American Academy of Pediatrics.

- Women of childbearing age should take a folic acid supplement before conception and up to the twelfth week of pregnancy.

- Pregnant women and nursing mothers should consider a vitamin D supplement and possibly an iron supplement if their iron levels are low.

- For all infants, children, and adolescents, beginning in the first few days of life, the American Academy of Pediatrics recommends a vitamin D intake of 400 IU per day, to prevent rickets and possibly to help with immunity and disease prevention. Talk to your child's doctor about whether your child should be taking a vitamin D supplement or any other supplements.

- Frail older people who have low caloric needs may benefit from a low-dose, balanced multivitamin.

- Older people should consider taking a vitamin D supplement, as should people who rarely go outdoors; people who cover up all their skin with clothes or sunscreen when outdoors, and those who don't eat meat or oily fish. Vitamin D levels can be tested by your doctor to determine if supplementation is necessary. An easy way to increase your levels is to allow yourself ten minutes, at least three days a week, of direct sunlight (no sunscreen) on your arms and legs. Studies are finding that a lot of people are low in vitamin D due to lack of direct sunlight exposure.

- If you are not getting adequate calcium and/or vitamin D, you may benefit from supplementation, especially if you are over fifty and at risk for osteoperosis.

- For patients with established heart disease, the American Heart Association recommends talking to their doctor about taking an omega-3 or fish oil supplement. The evidence is looking so promising that I take one every day even though I don't have known heart disease.

- People with low HDL ("good") cholesterol may benefit from a niacin supplement.

- If you want to take a multivitamin as insurance, like I do, there is little evidence of either benefit or harm. It probably can't hurt and might give your body nutrients it misses when you don't eat the foods you should. Talk it over with your doctor. My reason for taking it is probably more placebo than anything: I like to start my day feeling like I'm putting something good in my body, and along with a fish oil supplement, it's a better way to start my day than by eating a doughnut!

- If you are low in a particular vitamin or mineral or are suffering from certain medical conditions, your doctor may suggest supplementation for your individual circumstances.

- Lastly, remember: research is ever changing and we all have a lot more to learn about vitamin supplements!

ASK DR. STORK

Question: Are the so-called functional food ingredients of probiotics and prebiotics beneficial to my health?

Answer: Probiotics are "friendly" bacteria, or beneficial live microorganisms that are similar to those in the human gut. Foods that can contain probiotics include yogurt, miso, fermented and unfermented milk, and some soy drinks and juices.

Right now, probiotics are very popular, and when present in or added to foods, yogurts, and drinks, or taken in pill form, some believe they will do things like boost our immune system, regulate our digestive health, and help naturally strengthen the body's defenses. (A related but different concept is prebiotics, which are short-chain carbohydrates thought to improve the composition or metabolism of gut bacteria.)

The research on probiotics and health is in its infancy. According to a 2005 conference convened by the American Society of Microbiology, there is "some encouraging evidence" from the study of different specific probiotic formulations in these directions:

- To treat diarrhea, especially for diarrhea from rotavirus
- To prevent and treat infections of the urinary tract or female genital tract
- To treat irritable bowel syndrome
- To reduce recurrence of bladder cancer
- To shorten how long an intestinal infection lasts that is caused by a bacterium called *Clostridium difficile*
- To prevent and treat pouchitis, a condition that can follow surgery to remove part of the colon
- To prevent and manage atopic dermatitis (eczema) in children

Some major caveats: the experts found that in research of probiotics as cures, the benefits were usually low, a strong placebo effect occurs frequently, and more research is necessary to draw firm conclusions on probiotic effectiveness. Also, the safety of probiotics has not been studied thoroughly, and more information is needed, especially on young children, elderly people, and people with compromised immune systems.

Side effects tend to be mild, such as gas or bloating, but there could be as-yet-unknown unhealthy side effects to probiotics, including the theoretical risks of causing infections (especially in people with underlying health conditions) or overstimulation of the immune system.

I happen to love yogurt. I think it's good for overall health and I eat it often. When I see patients with diarrhea, especially after taking antibiotics, I often suggest they add yogurt with live cultures to their diet.

The Bottom Line: While major health benefits are not conclusively proven as of yet, I believe the evidence for probiotics is mounting and it's going to eventually be proven that including them in your diet is beneficial. I have added yogurt to my diet and you may want to consider adding foods like yogurt with live cultures to your overall healthy eating patterns.

Alternative: Herbal Supplements

What's not to love about herbal supplements?

They're all-natural products derived from those absolute miracles of cosmic engineering—plants, leaves, seeds, stems, bark, roots, and flowers. Based on thousands of years of folk wisdom and traditional medical knowledge, not only are they gifts from Mother Nature, but herbs have formed the basis of at least one third of all pharmaceutical drugs. Herbs are reported to help treat a dazzling array of ailments as diverse as insomnia, fatigue, depression, anxiety, enlarged prostate, obesity, dementia, and high blood pressure, and you can stroll into any health food store and buy them without a prescription. Sounds too good to be true, so it's little wonder that up to 25 percent of Americans report taking an herbal product in the last year, choosing from a vast selection of roughly 20,000 products available on the market totaling over $4 billion in sales. I've certainly tried some of them.

So I ask you, what's not to love about them?

Well, I'll give you four big reasons why you shouldn't blindly love them:

1. There is little solid proof that most herbal products actually work. That's not to say they absolutely don't work, but that there's little strong, consistent evidence yet that they do work.

2. Herbal products are subject to very little government regulation. Herbal manufacturers don't need to prove their products work before they sell them, unlike pharmaceutical companies. Sure, the drug companies are far from perfect, but herbal manufacturers have far less evidence to support their products.

3. Herbal products are sold with widely different amounts of ingredients and quality control, making it hard for the consumer to figure out exactly what they're buying.

4. There are safety concerns linked to a number of herbal products, most of which have not been rigorously tested on humans. Some herbal products are flat-out dangerous.

In 2008, Stephen Bent, MD, of the University of California, San Francisco Osher Center for Integrative Medicine, wrote an excellent paper in the *Journal of General Internal Medicine* (titled "Herbal Medicine in the United States") that gives the best bottom-line assessment of herbs that I've seen so far. Before you spend your hard-earned cash on an herbal product, or fall for the sales pitch of a vitamin shop salesperson, take a close look at Dr. Brent's point of view: "It is clear that there is limited evidence to support the efficacy of even the top ten herbs, and there is far less evidence for the remaining 20,000. This lack of evidence does not indicate a lack of benefit, but primarily indicates a lack of conclusive studies, positive or negative, for the efficacy of most herbal products." He added, "unfortunately, the true frequency of side effects for most herbs is not known because most have not been tested in large clinical trials and because surveillance systems are much less extensive than those in place for pharmaceutical products."

I believe that future research is going to show us that some herbs do amazing things for our health. In the meantime, we have a long way to go when it comes to rigorously studying most herbs. With some exceptions, the health benefits of most herbal products are understudied and their safety is largely unknown. Discuss specifics with your doctor. Remember, your doctor should be open-minded regarding herbs, but at the same time should only support using herbs that are safe and have some proven benefit for your condition.

Don't assume that just because you can pick something up in a health food store or vitamin shop that it's automatically safe. It is absolutely crucial that you tell your doctor about any herbs you are taking because some have the potential to interact and interfere with your medications and some may even increase bleeding during surgery. And remember, new studies and evidence are always emerging, so continue a dialogue with your doctor about herbs. You can follow ongoing research on herbs on the National Center for Complementary and Alternative Medicine's website: http://nccam.nih.gov.

Alternative: Detoxing

Walk into any health food store and you'll see shelves full of expensive potions, powders, and capsules promising to "cleanse your system" and remove deadly toxins that allegedly accumulate in your colon and cause all kinds of health problems.

But there's one big problem with this: the popular idea of "detoxing" and "cleansing" has no good science behind it.

It seems as if every January we are bombarded with detox articles in magazines and interviews with Hollywood celebrities gushing about how clean, pure, and happy they feel after a juice fast or a twenty-one-day cleanse or a coffee enema regimen. I heard of one detox plan that costs $350 for twenty-one days of powdered shakes. For the most part, these products have no compelling evidence to support their claims. They may have anecdotes, or theories, or a claim of tapping into ancient wisdom, but there's no medical support to back it up.

People can feel sharper and more energetic for a while after a so-called detox or cleanse, but it's probably because they've curtailed bad food habits, not because of anything that's unique to the powder, potion, or pill they've shelled out their hard-earned cash for. If someone feels better because they are eating healthier and/or consuming a more reasonable amount of calories, that's absolutely fantastic. That's exactly what should happen. The same goes for when people get regular physical activity. Rather than spend your money on a detox product or plan, you should find ways of adopting healthy behaviors into your lifestyle so you can stick to them for the long term, like Eating to Savor Life and enjoying a Daily Physical Vacation. There is simply no good science behind detoxing. The average human body does not accumulate deadly toxins in the colon or intestines that can be "flushed out" with a potion, powder, or overly restrictive diet that no one can stick to for more than a few weeks, maximum. Furthermore, your body does not need to be detoxified unless you are suffering from an acute poisoning, or another medical condition, in which case you should head straight to a hospital, not a health food store. Many of us do suffer from food abuse, in the sense that we eat very unhealthy, unbalanced diets, but the answer to that is simple: healthy eating, consuming a reasonable amount of calories, and regular physical activity—not a pill.

The medical fact is that you have a masterpiece detox system already at your fingertips. It is your own body. Twenty-four hours a day, your immune system, skin, respiratory system, kidneys, bloodstream, intestines, and liver all work together in magnificent cosmic harmony to protect you from dangerous substances, fight off viruses and bacteria, and filter out waste.

The Bottom Line: If you want to get your body's natural detox working more efficiently, follow the plan below. It is based on evidence, not hype:

DR. STORK'S ALL-NATURAL DETOX PLAN

The Top 7 Most Effective Ways to Support Your Body's Self-Cleansing Power and Boost Your Immune System

- Eat to Savor Life: engage in overall healthy eating patterns over the long term.
- Consume a sensible amount of calories, and limit "bad" fats and sodium.
- Get regular physical activity.
- Consume adequate fluids through the day (and I'm not talking about coffee and alcohol, folks!).
- If you consume alcohol, do so only in moderation.
- Do not use tobacco.
- Get adequate sleep.

DETOX STRATEGIES TO BE WARY OF

- Detox kits sold in health food stores.
- Detox and cleansing pills, powders, capsules, shakes, and dietary supplements.

- Detox plans based on overly restrictive diets that cut out meals or entire food groups.
- Enemas and laxatives, unless prescribed by your doctor.
- Vitamin and herbal supplements or other products claiming to detox your system.

Alternative: Acupuncture

I'd heard good things about the concept of acupuncture from others who had tried it, and I was curious. One day I went to the office of a skilled acupuncture practitioner who also happened to be a friend, lay back in a comfortable chair, and was intrigued as I watched her go to work inserting tiny sterile needles thought to stimulate well-being at key spots on and around my ears. Within minutes, something remarkable happened—I started experiencing feelings of warmth, energy, and peace ripple through my body. Maybe it was endorphins being released—but whatever it was, it was extraordinary. Today I often encourage my patients to consider acupuncture as a potential treatment for acute or chronic low back pain or other chronic pain if standard treatments haven't helped them, because there's good evidence to support it.

Acupuncture has been a pillar of traditional Chinese medicine for centuries and is used today for a broad spectrum of health conditions, especially for pain. The most common form of acupuncture is the penetration of the skin by needles at specific points thought to affect the flow of flow of "qi" (pronounced "chee"), or vital energy, along passageways called meridians. Millions of people swear by acupuncture, and use it to help relieve pain in the back, joints, and neck, and for headaches, osteoarthritis, tennis elbow, postoperative dental pain, carpal tunnel syndrome, fibromyalgia, and menstrual cramps.

The fascinating thing about acupuncture is that it actually works for some people with certain types of pain, but it is next to impossible for so-called Western medicine to definitively explain why it may work. Some experts argue that acupuncture helps activate pain-relieving chemicals like endorphins at key locations in the body—in other words, acupuncture is thought to enable your body to release its own natural painkillers. But when acupuncture is rigorously tested against so-called sham acupuncture or placebo acupuncture, which involves needling at the wrong points, both techniques often produce some relief in pain. This suggests that other forces are also at work, like perhaps the enthusiastic expectations of the patient and the close bonding and positive focus shared by practitioner and patient that's typical of acupuncture sessions. In essence, psychological forces may be creating or enhancing a biological effect. (I definitely felt something in my mind and my body when I had acupuncture many years ago.)

On the plus side, the National Center for Complementary and Alternative Medicine points out that a 2008 review of clinical trials published in the *British Journal of Anaesthesia* noted that acupuncture has value for reducing postoperative pain. The organization also notes that both the American College of Physicians and the American Pain Society have issued clinical guidelines supporting acupuncture as a treatment option for chronic back pain. And as published in the December 2004 edition of *Annals of Internal Medicine*, one of the biggest randomized clinical trials of acupuncture ever conducted found that acupuncture provided significant pain relief and improved function for people with osteoarthritis of the knee, as compared to both sham acupuncture and a control group that received counseling only.

There is some preliminary evidence that acupuncture given as a complement to in vitro fertilization, or IVF, can increase the odds of achieving pregnancy, and that acupuncture may help people with post-traumatic stress disorder, or PTSD. Acupuncture can be an effective treatment for headaches as well. Duke researchers, after analyzing data from seventeen studies, found acupuncture to be effective for treating those who suffer from migraine headaches: 62 percent of those receiving acupuncture reported relief versus 45 percent of those taking medication.

When performed properly by an experienced practitioner using sterile needles, acupuncture is generally considered safe. Adverse reactions are rare but include infections.

My Opinion: Acupuncture is a fascinating complement to conventional treatments, as it may offer you pain relief, especially for back pain, headaches, or osteoarthritis; and might aid in IVF treatments. Just don't expect miracles, and realize that benefits might also flow from your own positive feelings. Then again, there is absolutely nothing wrong with feeling better physically and having positive feelings!

Talk to your doctor about acupuncture if you're interested. I suggest you obtain an acupuncture referral from your medical doctor or someone you trust, because just like any type of medicine, you want to go to someone who knows what they are doing and who practices sterile techniques.

Alternative: Reiki

Reiki, pronounced "ray-kee," is a healing technique that started in Japan, and involves a Reiki practitioner putting their hands lightly on, or just above, your body in key spots in hopes of boosting the body's natural healing power.

Many claims and testimonials have been made for Reiki as a complementary treatment, including:

- Promoting overall health and well-being.

- Boosting the immune system.

- Offering relief from disease symptoms and medical treatment side effects.

- Aiding in relaxation, and reducing anxiety and stress.

- Relieving chronic pain, allergies, high blood pressure, and heart conditions.

- Helping terminally ill patients and their families and caregivers achieve peace.

These claims have not been well substantiated yet by medical research. A major review of Reiki research published in 2008 in the *International Journal of Clinical Practice* ("Effects of reiki in clinical practice: a systematic review of randomised clinical trials") concluded that "the evidence is insufficient to suggest that Reiki is an effective treatment for any condition," and "the value of reiki remains unproven." But the fact is that many people genuinely enjoy and seem to derive real benefits from Reiki sessions, which do not have major risks or side effects when performed properly, and many patients and increasingly many doctors and nurses are so intrigued by the potential of Reiki as an adjunct to traditional care that it is popping up in medical offices, hospitals, and clinics around the United States. For example, at the Cleveland Clinic, one of the nation's most well-respected mainstream medical institutions, Reiki is being studied for its impact on anxiety and prostate cancer, and at George Washington University Medical Center in Washington, D.C., Dr. Joel Rosenberg, director of clinical cardiology, has launched a Reiki program for patients, their families, and staff members to help them reduce stress. He told the *Washington Post* that pain scores go down three or four points on a ten-point scale after Reiki sessions, reductions occur in heart rates, and sedation and inflammation decrease.

I personally had a Reiki session to try it out and it did absolutely nothing for me, but again, alternative therapy is about figuring out what is safe and what may work for you. Just because it doesn't work for me doesn't mean Reiki won't work for you, and at least it is safe.

My Opinion: Reiki is so far an unproven treatment, but it appears to have potential to safely reduce stress and foster relaxation, especially in a medical environment, with low risk.

Alternative: Chiropractic

If you want to start a hot debate, get some doctors and chiropractors in a room and have them talk about chiropractic treatments.

Some medical doctors and researchers see chiropractic care as effective for certain conditions, but others see chiropractic as a worthless treatment, a waste of money, and a potentially counterproductive detour for a patient when they should be getting regular medical care. For example, a major research review published in 2008 in the *Journal of Pain and Symptom Management* found that "the concepts of chiropractic are not based on solid science," and "with the possible exception of back pain, chiropractic spinal manipulation has not been shown to be effective for any medical condition."

Personally, I have some great friends who are chiropractors and I see the potential for chiropractic to help as a complement in certain conditions. Plus, many millions of Americans swear by it as an alternative treatment.

According to the NCCAM, here's what we know about chiropractic care from the evidence gathered so far:

- Patients report very high levels of satisfaction with chiropractic care.

- Overall, studies of spinal manipulation show minimal to moderate evidence of short-term relief of back pain. Information on cost-effectiveness, dosing, and long-term benefit is scant.

- Although clinical trials have found no evidence that spinal manipulation is an effective treatment for asthma, hypertension, or dysmenorrhea, spinal manipulation may be as effective as some medications for both migraine and tension headaches and may offer short-term benefits to those suffering from neck pain.

- There are some risks associated with manipulation of the spine, but most reported side effects have been mild and of short duration. Although rare, incidents of stroke and vertebral artery dissection have been reported following manipulation of the cervical spine.

My Opinion: If your back pain doesn't respond well to conservative treatments and your doctor has ruled out fractures, malignancy, and other life-threatening causes of your pain, chiropractic treatments are an option to consider.

Alternative: Massage Therapy

Massage therapy may be the most ancient and universal of all alternative treatments, dating back to ancient India, Arabia, Egypt, Greece, and Rome.

A recent survey found that some 18 million adults and 700,000 children in America had received massage therapy in the previous year for general health and wellness and for specific conditions like pain, sports injuries, stress, anxiety, and depression. There are lots of different kinds of massage therapy, including Swedish massage, reflexology, shiatsu, Rolfing, and craniosacral therapy.

Does it work?

The research is not open-and-shut, but there are good theories and some good evidence to support massage therapy. It's possible that massage may trigger the release of body chemicals like endorphins and serotonin, and may block pain signals traveling to the brain. One session of massage therapy may decrease anxiety, heart rate, and blood pressure, and a series of treatments may help alleviate depression and pain. The most promising area in which massage therapy may be effective is in the treatment of low-back pain. In my experience, massage is also very helpful in the rehabilitation of certain sports injuries.

It looks like massage therapy has few major risks if it is administered properly by a trained professional. The National Certification Board for Therapeutic Massage & Bodywork (NCBTMB) certifies practitioners who pass a national test. Increasingly, the many states that license massage therapists require them to have at least five hundred hours of training at an accredited institution, pass the NCBTMB exam, have malpractice insurance, and fulfill specific continuing education requirements.

My Opinion: Massage therapy is a promising treatment for pain management and relaxation and is generally thought to have few adverse effects.

Check with your doctor before starting massage therapy if you have a medical condition, especially pregnancy, bleeding disorders, low blood platelet counts, blood clots, fractures, open or healing wounds, skin infections, weakened bones (such as from osteoporosis or cancer), a recent surgery, a cancerous tumor, or if you're taking blood-thinning medications like warfarin.

Alternative: Homeopathy

As a medical doctor, homeopathy makes very little sense to me.

Homeopathy is based on a theory that a disease can be cured by a substance that produces similar symptoms in healthy people, and that the body's healing systems can be enhanced by introducing the substance into the body in a very diluted form.

The theory behind standard vaccinations is based on roughly similar logic, but homeopathy is based on dilutions so extreme that their effectiveness lacks any plausible explanation in modern science, physics, or chemistry.

I know there are many people who are passionate about their homeopathic remedies (a recent survey estimated that almost 4 million adults and 900,000 children used homeopathy in the previous year), and you can find countless homeopathic products in health food stores and on the internet, with mountains of testimonials and anecdotes to back them up as cures for many illnesses. But these are stories, not scientific evidence.

There are rare studies that suggest a benefit for homeopathy above that of the placebo effect, but there is little conclusive, consistent evidence supporting the use of homeopathy for any medical condition, which has led much of the medical and scientific community to dismiss it out of hand. The NCCAM has this to say about side effects of homeopathy:

- The side effects and risks of homeopathic treatments are not well researched, but a systematic review found that homeopathic remedies in high dilution, taken under the supervision of trained professionals, are generally considered safe and unlikely to cause severe adverse reactions.

- Liquid homeopathic remedies may contain alcohol. The FDA allows higher levels of alcohol in these remedies than it allows in conventional drugs. However, no adverse effects from alcohol levels have been reported to the FDA.

- Homeopaths expect some of their patients to experience homeopathic aggravation (a temporary worsening of existing symptoms after taking a homeopathic prescription). Researchers have not found much evidence of this reaction in clinical studies; however, research on homeopathic aggravations is scarce.

- Homeopathic remedies are not known to interfere with conventional drugs; however, if you are considering using homeopathic remedies, you should discuss this with your health care provider first.

- There is currently no uniform licensing or professional standards for the practice of homeopathy in the United States; the licensing of homeopaths varies from state to state.

My Opinion: Any benefits of homeopathy could very well be the result of the patient's positive mind-set and expectations for the homeopathic product, as well as bonding well with the practitioner, rather than any significant biological effect of the product itself. A homeopathic remedy alone probably has a low risk of hurting you, but you're taking a risk if you use a homeopathic product as a substitute for qualified medical attention.

If you absolutely love homeopathy, you're probably not doing any harm, so I would never tell you to stop using it. It is difficult for me to recommend it, however, unless good evidence for it emerges, like a pattern of positive randomized clinical trials.

ASK DR. STORK

Question: I'm hearing more and more about resveratrol—what is it, and does it really slow down the aging process?

Answer: Resveratrol is an antioxidant found in Concord grapes, red wine, blueberries, and other fruits. Based on research conducted on animals, it is believed that resveratrol might help resist the aging process, in part by increasing the activity of sirtuins, or proteins that function like enzymes to help cells resist stress. Resveratrol may also help reduce inflammation and have anti-cancer effects.

Resveratrol supplements have exploded into a huge mini-industry thanks to a positive *60 Minutes* TV report a few years ago and an explosion of internet hype and scams that followed a mention of resveratrol on *The Oprah Winfrey Show*. But the problem with resveratrol is that it has not been at all well studied in humans, and the case for any benefits it has on human aging or other conditions is purely speculative and theoretical at this point in time.

The Bottom Line: Get resveratrol in your diet the all-natural way, with dark Concord grapes, blueberries, and, if you enjoy wine, a glass of red wine. I say a glass, because moderation is essential if you want a positive health benefit. Anything beyond a glass a day for women, or two for men, can actually start placing your health in jeopardy regardless of how much resveratrol is in your system.

The benefits of resveratrol supplements are completely unproven so far in humans, and the side effects of resveratrol supplements in humans are unknown, so stay tuned for further research.

---

7 QUICK, ALTERNATIVE TIPS TO MAKE YOUR HOME HEALTHIER

One alternative health idea that many people forget about is a toxin-free house. You may not know it, but your home may be making you sick.

We spend about 90 percent of our lives indoors, and the majority of that time is in our own homes. When was the last time you stopped to think about the harmful or toxic chemicals, pollutants, and other substances that may have set up camp in your house? They could be giving you a cough, irritating your eyes, or, as a worst case, they could be increasing your risk for illnesses like lung cancer.

Most people don't need to spend thousands of dollars to "detox" their home; a few simple things can make a big difference. Here are seven quick and easy steps you can take to make your home a healthier place:

1. Test your home for radon.

Radon is a radioactive invisible gas that is present in some homes. It comes from the soil and from some granite fixtures and it causes about 21,000 deaths from lung cancer each year in the United States, second only to tobacco use.

No matter where you live in the United States, it's a good idea to have your home tested for radon. You can buy an inexpensive testing kit for around $20, or hire an expert to do the testing for you.

For excellent information on radon resources in your area, go to: http://www.epa.gov/radon.

2. Control the mold.

Molds are natural organisms that occur almost everywhere, and they thrive indoors, especially in damp conditions. Mold is usually not a major health risk, but exposure to too much mold in the home can worsen asthma and is linked to upper respiratory symptoms, like nasal irritation and coughing. So if someone in your family is suffering from one of these symptoms, mold could be the culprit.

Take time to regularly clean up the mold that often collects on bathroom and kitchen surfaces. Remember, mold can grow behind and in between walls, so it's not always going to be visible. For bigger mold problems, call in a professional for an inspection and cleanup.

3. Buy a water filter.

Tap water is, in my opinion, superior to most bottled water. Why? Because it's supercheap. It doesn't harm the environment like plastic bottles do, and many bottled water companies won't even disclose basic information about their water, but public water systems are highly regulated by the government. Tap water also is fluoridated, which is good for our teeth. And believe it or not, the bottled water you are drinking may just be tap water in disguise.

I drink tap water all the time. I use a BPA-free reusable water bottle and fill it every day with cold tap water before I leave home for work. Tap water isn't perfect, though; the Associated Press did an analysis in 2008 of samples from around the United States and found trace amounts of many unexpected chemicals and drugs in the water supply, including antibiotics and antidepressants. And in late 2009 the nonprofit organization Environmental Working Group did a major analysis of the tests on the nation's tap water and found pollutants in the water supplies of many metropolitan areas, though usually not in violation of any legal standards, which themselves may unfortunately be outdated.

If you're concerned about the quality of your tap water, get a good water filter. They can filter out everything from lead to chlorine, and you can get them for around $20 at many stores.

And check out the www.ewg.org website for city-by-city tap water test results and tips on buying a water filter.

4. Dial down the BPA.

Bisphenol A, or BPA, is an ingredient found in plastic bottles, baby bottles, and metal food cans. Some research suggests that BPA is an endocrine-disrupting chemical that can "leach out" of the bottle into food and beverages, and may increase rates of prostate cancer, breast cancer, and reproductive problems.

The National Toxicology Program has reported "some concern" for BPA's effects on the brain, behavior, and prostate gland in fetuses, infants, and children, at current human exposures to BPA. For people who are concerned about BPA, the National Institutes of Health suggests these steps:

- Don't microwave polycarbonate plastic food containers. Polycarbonate is strong and durable, but over time it may break down from overuse at high temperatures. Polycarbonate containers that contain BPA usually have a "7" on the bottom.
- Reduce your use of canned foods or make sure the can is BPA free.

- When possible, opt for glass, porcelain, or stainless steel containers, particularly for hot food or liquids.
- Use baby bottles and plastic bottles that are BPA free.

5. Use a HEPA vacuum cleaner at least once a week.

Our homes, and especially our carpets, can become heavily polluted with largely invisible concentrations of dust, dust mites, cat and dog dander, and other icky debris. These irritants can aggravate allergies, upper respiratory infections, and asthma, for which children are especially vulnerable.

To reduce these concentrations, use a high-efficiency particulate air (HEPA) vacuum cleaner at least once a week, and spend extra time vacuuming your carpets. HEPA vacuum cleaners are superior to standard vacuum cleaners for removing allergens and benefiting respiratory health in asthmatic children.

6. Use simple, gentle cleaning products.

In twentieth century America we fell victim to the idea that more and more chemicals made us healthier. The cleaner, the better, we thought, and the more powerful and specialized the cleaner, the better the result. We developed scrubbing bubble foam for our toilets. Tub and tile cleaners for one purpose, and spray aerosols for another. Glass cleaners, all-purpose cleaners, rug cleaners—you name it, we cleaned with it.

The result is that we loaded up our homes with some of the most disgusting smells and overpowering chemical compounds we could dream up. Did you ever notice how many of these products warn us in capital letters to ventilate the room or use extreme caution? Hey, that probably means we shouldn't have this stuff in our houses!

The fact is, we simply do not know what the long-term impact of all these specialized, powerful chemicals will have on our health. I doubt it's good. It's a mystery as to how these toxins interact with each other. For example, it's troubling to me how autoimmune illnesses seem to be on the rise in America and we don't know why. There is a theory that we have so many chemicals and antibacterials around the house that our own immune systems are becoming less efficient.

I think that there are good arguments that the more natural cleaning products we use, and the fewer harsh chemicals, the safer we'll be in the long run, and it will also be better for the environment. I don't like bleach or ammonia, which can irritate my eyes and make it difficult to breathe, so I've converted in my own home to all-natural cleaning products. Unfortunately there are no consistent standards yet for all-natural cleaning products, so I look for items mainly consisting of things like peroxide, baking soda, vinegar, and simple soaps, and search for products with the shortest ingredient lists possible.

Play it safe: clean your home with simple, environmentally conscious products that have as few harsh chemicals as possible—especially if you have young kids running around the house.

7. Never allow any kind of smoking in your house.

Smoking not only can kill the smoker; the smoker's family members can become victims of secondhand smoke. Living with a smoker has been linked to a 20 percent higher risk of developing lung cancer and a 25 percent higher risk of coronary artery disease. In children, environmental tobacco smoke is linked to sudden infant death syndrome, childhood respiratory problems and other illnesses.

The bottom line is obvious—no smoking in the house, ever—period!

ASK DR. STORK

Question: If I do catch a cold, what should I do?

Answer: The first thing to do is drink plenty of fluids (and I don't mean alcohol!) and Eat to Savor Life. Your body and immune system need nutrients to fight off infection and speed recovery.

If you're using over-the-counter medications like cough syrup, nasal spray, or a pain reliever, realize that they are for symptomatic treatment only and will not reduce the duration of a cold. They can also have side effects—overuse of decongestant nasal sprays for more than a few days, for example, can cause dependence and "rebound" effects that can make the problem worse.

You should also realize that many cold remedies contain multiple ingredients you may not be aware of, like acetaminophen. So if you double up on over-the-counter meds, you may very well unknowingly be taking the same ingredient in multiple doses, putting yourself at risk for adverse effects. In the case of acetaminophen, if you are accidentally ingesting more than the recommended amount, it can lead to liver damage. So remember to read the ingredients!

Currently, there is no cure for the common cold other than time. Colds are caused by viruses, not bacteria, so antibiotics are completely worthless. In fact, taking antibiotics when we don't need them increases bacterial resistance and makes antibiotics less effective when we really do need them.

ASK DR. STORK

Question: What do you think about using a neti pot?

Answer: The next time you're congested, try using a neti pot.

The neti pot looks like a little teapot. It's a simple, nonaddictive, effective treatment for relieving nasal congestion, sinusitis, and nasal symptoms of allergies and the common cold. You fill it with saline to clean out your sinuses of clogging mucus, bacteria, and viral and allergic particles. The process is called nasal irrigation. Unlike nasal decongestants, there's no "rebound effect." And there's good research that indicates that the neti pot works.

I use a neti pot almost every day, especially when I'm in Los Angeles, where I find the air can be really irritating. It also helps to keep my seasonal allergy symptoms in check. You can pick up a neti pot at almost any drug store for as little as $10, including the packs of saline solution. (If you don't like the idea of using a neti pot, a simpler method is to use saline spray, which is also available at any drugstore.)

Open Your Mind to Alternatives: Quick and Easy Takeaway

- You should be as open-minded and yet as tough on alternative medicine as you should be on mainstream medicine—demand the evidence! It is your right and your duty as a patient and as a consumer.

- The most effective alternative medicines are healthy eating and regular physical activity.

- With a few exceptions, the health benefits of most vitamin and herbal supplements are currently not proven. It's usually best to get your nutrients from healthy eating patterns.

- Acupuncture, chiropractic care, and massage are promising complementary treatment options for some pain conditions, especially musculoskeletal back pain. Reiki is unproven as of yet but is gaining strong interest in the medical community.

- Homeopathic remedies are generally unproven.

- Tell your doctor, dentist, and surgeon about any alternative medicine or therapies you are taking—some can have serious adverse effects on your prescription medicines and can even cause surgical complications like excess bleeding.

- Some good resources for following new developments in alternative medicine are:
  http://nccam.nih.gov
  www.pubmed.com
  www.webmd.com
  www.mayoclinic.com
  www.quackwatch.org

- Benefits of many alternative treatments may largely be driven by the patient's positive mind-set. And that is absolutely okay.

- Keep an open mind to all the evidence. New research is coming out all the time, and expert opinions can change.

- Last but not least, if it sounds too good to be true, it probably is!

SEVEN

MAKE THE MIND-BODY CONNECTION

"You are a father," the nurse whispered as she lay the newborn infant down gently on the man's chest. This is normally an incredibly joyous occasion—the first time a man meets his child.

But in this case it was a tragic scene—the forty-one-year-old man, John, was in a coma, stretched out in a hospital bed. At the same time his thirty-two-year-old wife Connie had given birth, John, a police-man in New Jersey, was in the hospital after suffering an aortic dis-section, which occurs when the inner wall of the aorta rips open and blood pours through. It is a massive cardiac emergency and death can occur within minutes or seconds. John underwent a five-and-a-half-hour surgery to repair the tear in his aortic wall. During the ordeal, the normally vibrant police officer flatlined. He suffered multiorgan failure and a stroke. Then he fell into an unconscious state with little immediate hope in sight.

The infant brushed against the man's chest, and breathed on his father's face.

Then something happened that stunned everybody in the room: the policeman opened his eyes.

In that moment, feeling the warm presence of his child, John snapped out of his semiconscious state and began his long recovery.

The three of them—Connie, John, and their gorgeous son Levi—all appeared on *The Doctors,* and I, along with our entire audience, was profoundly moved by their story. Think about it: something happened inside John's brain that was so beautiful that it shattered the spell of a terrible physical condition, liberating his mind and his body, giving him a new chance at life. All from a baby's breath and something completely mysterious that happened inside John's mind.

This family's story reminded me how medical miracles happen every day, all the time, all around the world. Magnificent things happen to people's health that simply can't be explained by modern science. It also reminded me how important the power of love and hope are to the process of health and wellness, and how little we really know about the potential of the human spirit to conquer illness.

Ultimately, it reminded me that the connection between the mind and the body is perhaps the most powerful yet least understood force when it comes to our health.

I can't explain to you why John woke up out of his coma. Nobody can. We can't always explain why there's such a unique connection between the power of the mind over the body, but just because we can't explain or measure it doesn't mean it doesn't exist. On the contrary.

I've seen so many miracles happen in the hospital. I've seen patients with terrible injuries heal unexpectedly. I've seen children "come back from the dead" and talk vividly about the experience. I've seen adults who have been at death's door with multiple chronic diseases make their minds up to change their lifestyle and master their destiny, and they've totally turned their lives and their health around in a positive direction.

I've seen patients achieve miracles that no drug could possibly accomplish.

The ability of your mind to influence your health may be the most promising road to optimal wellness we have.

I am an unapologetic believer in the mind-body connection, and in this chapter I'll explore how to harness the power of this phenomenon.

GREAT NEWS: WHAT THE EVIDENCE TELLS US ABOUT THE MIND-BODY CONNECTION

Mind-body concepts have long been a part of Indian, Chinese, and other world traditions of healing, and they are now moving into the mainstream of Western medicine.

Mind-body medicine focuses on the powerful ways that emotional, mental, and spiritual forces can directly impact our health. The scientific study of mind-body medicine is a relatively new field, and it includes subjects as diverse as meditation, yoga, prayer, hypnosis, biofeedback, relaxation, guided imagery, spirituality, and art, music, and dance therapies. The research reveals some great news: mind-body therapies can really work!

According to the National Center for Complementary and Alternative Medicine (NCCAM) and a review by experts at the Harvard Medical School Osher Research Center published in the June 2009 issue of the *Journal of Psychosomatic Research* ("Alternative mind-body therapies used by adults with medical conditions"), here are the research headlines:

- Patients report high rates (68 to 90 percent) of perceived helpfulness for mind-body therapies for specific medical conditions.

- Mind-body therapies are used by 16.6 percent of adults in the United States.

- Mind-body interventions have positive effects on psychological functioning and quality of life.

- The brain and the central nervous system may influence immune, endocrine, and autonomic functioning, which are known to have an impact on health.

- Mind-body approaches can be effective supporting treatments for coronary artery disease and pain-related disorders like arthritis and a variety of other chronic conditions.

- Mind-body therapies used before surgery can improve recovery time and reduce pain after the procedure.

- The physical and emotional risks of most mind-body interventions are minimal.

- Most mind-body interventions, when tested and standardized, can easily be taught.

- The evidence for benefits for certain indications from biofeedback, cognitive-behavioral interventions, and hypnosis is quite good, and there is emerging evidence regarding their physiological effects. There is less research supporting the use of meditation and yoga, but that doesn't mean they aren't effective.

- Evidence from multiple studies with various types of cancer patients suggests that mind-body interventions can improve mood, quality of life, and coping, as well as ameliorate disease and treatment-related symptoms, such as chemotherapy-induced nausea, vomiting, and pain.

Let's have a look at some of the most interesting ways you can use the mind-body connection to optimize your health.

Mind-Body Connection: Yoga

I think there are very few people on Earth who wouldn't benefit from yoga. If you've never tried it, I urge you to consider it.

I love yoga. I'm not a yoga buff—I don't do it every day by any means, and there's much more I have to learn about it. But I've experienced both yoga and Bikram Yoga, also known as Hot Yoga, and

I've done Pilates, which is based in part on yoga. I really enjoy them all and wish I had time to do them more. Yoga delivers a wonderful range of feelings—after a yoga session, I always feel so calm and flexible and peaceful.

Yoga is a system of physical postures, breathing techniques, and meditation that's been around for thousands of years, and it is practiced today by some 12 million American adults and 1.5 million children. The Yoga Sutras, a text written in India more than two thousand years ago, outlined the spiritual foundations of yoga practice, things I think we all need more of in our stressed out, often chaotic modern world, including moral behavior, healthy habits, breathing exercises, and meditation.

There are many different kinds of yoga, and people use yoga for a wide range of purposes: for physical fitness, reducing stress and high blood pressure, relaxation, spiritual growth, anxiety disorders, and depression. Yoga also serves as a form of meditation.

While more well-designed studies are needed before definitive conclusions can be drawn about yoga's use for specific health conditions, here's how the National Center for Complementary and Alternative Medicine says yoga may help optimize our health, according to the evidence:

How Yoga May Help Optimize Health

- Improve overall physical fitness, strength, and flexibility.

- Enhance stress-coping mechanisms and mind-body awareness.

- Boost mood and feelings of well-being, reduce stress.

- Decrease blood pressure and heart rate.

- Boost lung capacity.

- Improve muscle relaxation and body composition.

- Provide benefits for conditions like insomnia, anxiety, and depression.

- Improve levels of beneficial blood and brain chemicals.

My Opinion: I highly recommend yoga. It's a great way to pamper your mind and body, reduce stress, and increase relaxation, and there is evidence that it can positively affect your health. All it takes is a mat and a class or instructional DVD.

Most forms of yoga are considered safe and present few side effects. However, some yoga practices and poses should be avoided by people with certain medical issues like pregnancy and osteoporosis, among others—so check with your doctor before you try it.

Mind-Body Connection: Meditation

I strongly believe in the power of meditation to help improve your mental and physical health.

Meditation means many things to many people. For some people it may simply mean deep breathing, for others prayer, and forms of meditation include mindfulness meditation, relaxation response, mantra meditation, and Zen Buddhist meditation. For me, meditation means anything you can do that takes your mind off of everything else and puts your mind at rest. Meditation techniques often feature a peaceful location free of distractions and a calming focus of attention, like a series of words or the rhythms of breathing.

I practice "active meditation," where I become so intensely focused on an activity that I'm blocking everything else out of my mind. I achieve this intense state of focus when I go mountain biking or white-water kayaking, and I believe it works wonders to reduce my stress levels. It also rejuvenates me mentally and physically. Other people may choose to follow a slower, more Zen-like approach to meditating while at rest or walking at an easy pace.

People use meditation as a routine part of their life to enjoy well-being, peace, and relaxation. They also use it to address conditions like insomnia, stress, depression, pain, and symptoms of chronic illnesses like HIV/AIDS or heart disease.

It is important to note that there is not much evidence yet that proves a direct positive impact of meditation upon health. Better research needs to be done. But I believe that the future will hold major evidence breakthroughs for the health benefits of meditation. So far, here's where the evidence on meditation is starting to lead us, in the words of the NCCAM.

How Meditation Might Work to Optimize Health

- Some types of meditation might work by affecting the autonomic (involuntary) nervous system. This system regulates many organs and muscles, controlling functions such as the heartbeat, sweating, breathing, and digestion. It has two major parts:

  - The sympathetic nervous system helps mobilize the body for action. When a person is under stress, it produces the fight-or-flight response: the heart rate and breathing rate go up and blood vessels narrow.

  - The parasympathetic nervous system does the opposite: it causes the heart rate and breathing rate to slow down, the blood vessels to dilate, and digestive juices to increase.

- It is thought that some types of meditation might work by reducing activity in the sympathetic nervous system and increasing activity in the parasympathetic nervous system.

- In one area of research, scientists are using sophisticated tools to determine whether meditation is associated with significant changes in brain function. A number of researchers believe that these changes account for many of meditation's effects.

- It is also possible that practicing meditation may work by improving the mind's ability to pay attention. Since attention is involved in performing everyday tasks and regulating mood, meditation might lead to other benefits.

- Meditation is considered to be safe for healthy people. There have been rare reports that meditation could cause or worsen symptoms in people who have certain psychiatric problems, but this question has not been fully researched.

My Opinion: Meditation techniques are promising concepts for reducing stress and aiding relaxation, therefore helping overall health and well-being.

If you're interested, you can look into many types of meditation practices and see which ones seem most beneficial for you.

DR. STORK'S STRESS BUSTER:
THE 5 DEEP BREATHS MEDITATION EXERCISE

One day my best friend and I were hiking deep in the wilderness along the Appalachian Trail. We were rushing to get through a four-day hike, and we were treating it like an endurance contest.

It was cool and crisp and the mountain air was intoxicating. The view was spectacular. Rain began to pour down. Suddenly, as I stood in the rain, I became overwhelmed by the feeling of pure, unadulterated nature all around me.

"Wait a minute," I said. "What the heck are we doing? Why are we in such a rush? Let's just take five deep breaths and enjoy this moment."

We did, and it felt wonderful. I experienced an instant feeling of contentment that was almost like an instant positive physical transformation. All the stresses of the hike and the pent-up pressures of my professional life just melted away in the cool rain.

From then on, Five Deep Breaths has become my mantra. I do it whenever I feel stressed, and I do it whenever I need to slow down. It almost always works.

We can go nuts from all the demands and distractions in our busy lives and forget to breathe deeply, and it's not good for our health. Here's what you can do to counteract the chaos:

Take five long, slow, relaxing deep breaths:

When you wake up in the morning.

When you go to sleep at night.

Whenever you feel stressed during the day.

Take a deep breath in, hold it for a few seconds, and then count slowly to ten while you exhale. It may be one of the easiest, cheapest, and most effective stress busters you've ever tried!

Mind-Body Connection: Tai Chi

Tai Chi is a Chinese practice also known as "moving meditation." The theory behind it is that it aids the flow of life energies in the body. Tai Chi combines relaxed deep breathing with slow, graceful body movements that reflect movements in animals and nature, such as Grasp the Bird's Tail and Embrace Tiger, Return to Mountain. In Chinese-American communities you can often see Tai Chi being practiced early in the morning in public parks.

I find Tai Chi a fascinating concept, as it combines elements of weight-bearing, low-impact aerobic exercise, posture, and flexibility with deep breathing and meditation, all of which I believe can greatly benefit our health.

People use Tai Chi for many reasons—for overall health and physical fitness, and for specific benefits like improving balance and preventing falls among senior citizens, relieving osteoarthritis pain, and promoting cardiovascular health. So far, most of the studies on Tai Chi have been small, inconclusive and/or not well designed. Much more research is needed before it can be recommended as clinically useful for specific medical conditions. But there are preliminary suggestions in the research that Tai Chi might:

- Enhance the immune system, cardiovascular fitness, and overall well-being in older people.

- Reduce falls and reduce blood pressure among older people.

- Help in pain control for patients with knee osteoarthritis.

- Help with lower extremity range of motion for people with rheumatoid arthritis.

Tai Chi is considered safe for healthy people, but if you have a medical condition, check with your doctor before doing Tai Chi or any other exercise. There is no standard training, licensing, or regulation for Tai Chi instructors, so you're pretty much on your own when choosing one.

My Opinion: Its health benefits are not yet clearly proven, but Tai Chi is a safe and very promising form of both exercise and meditation.

Mind-Body Connection: High-Quality Sleep

When we first started taping *The Doctors* in 2008, I moved to a partially furnished apartment in Los Angeles. Soon after, I started feeling really lousy.

I loved my new job and really enjoyed all the people I was working with. I liked the challenge of putting on a great show every day and communicating lifesaving and life-improving medical information to millions of people. But I'd never felt so stressed out before in my whole life. I was feeling a constant buzz of fatigue, and I couldn't figure out why. I was doing everything you're supposed to do to be healthy—living clean, exercising regularly, and eating really nutritious food most of the time. I just wasn't myself.

Why was I feeling so burned out?

At first I thought it was from the stress associated with being on national TV every day and figuring out how I was going to balance everything while continuing life as an ER doctor.

Then one day we taped a program segment about how mattresses affect how well you sleep. I lay down on a magnificent premium mattress on our stage, and it felt spectacular. I couldn't believe how comfortable I was. My whole body just relaxed, and I wanted to go to sleep right there on national TV!

I realized that one of the reasons I'd been feeling so lousy was because I wasn't sleeping well. And when I lay down on that mattress it hit me—I'd been sleeping on an uncomfortable, inferior mattress every night in LA, the type that bends in the middle and gives no support. No wonder I was tossing and turning all night. How could I have missed something so obvious that was so negatively affecting my overall health?

I purchased one of those mattresses and had it rushed to my place. Soon after I started enjoying some of the deepest, most refreshing and peaceful sleeps I've ever experienced. The type that only half a year of sleep deprivation can provide!

One of the most essential mind-body connections we can make is to get quality sleep, which means both the right amount of sleep and the right kind of sleep—preferably deep and very comfortable.

It's amazing how a good night's sleep can mean the difference between a productive day and one that's a struggle to get through, and something as simple as an old, uncomfortable, or dirty mattress or pillow can really foul up your sleeping without your even realizing it. Think about it—one third of your life is controlled by an object you lay your head down on every night, and that bed can screw up your life or enhance it. So invest in good bedding! If you are going to try to save money, I recommend paying a little less for a car and using the extra money to upgrade your mattress.

Stress can keep us from sleeping well, too, of course. Two-thirds of Americans say they lose sleep because of stress, and with a volatile economy, wars raging, and a steady diet of twenty-four-hour cable news, who can blame us? But despite the legitimate causes of our tossing and turning, we must do our best to combat them. Why? According to experts at Mental Health America (MHA), poor sleep has been linked to such major health problems as:

- Higher risk of depression and anxiety

- Higher risk of heart disease and cancer

- Impaired memory

- Reduced immune system functioning

- Weight gain

- Greater likelihood of accidents

Here are tips for cranking up the quality of your sleep, including tips courtesy of Mental Health America:

- Go to bed and wake up at a regular time—your body loves consistent sleep habits.

- Moderate your caffeine intake. Skip coffee after lunch.

- Exercise. Regular physical activity can improve your sleep by reducing stress and tension. Avoid exercising right before bed, though, since it may make you more alert and less sleepy.

- Destress yourself by taking a hot bath, reading, or doing something quiet and peaceful before you go to bed.

- Make your bed a quality sleep zone. Make sure you've got a comfortable mattress. Get the room dark and quiet. Don't pay bills, surf the net, or watch TV in bed. Try to relax and let go of stressful ideas.

- For more sleep tips, see the National Sleep Foundation's website, www.sleepfoundation.org.

- If you have persistent sleep problems, check with your doctor to rule out an underlying health problem. A sleep clinic or sleep therapist may help, for example, through cognitive-behavioral therapy for insomnia, which addresses sleep-related beliefs and behaviors.

3 EASY, EVERYDAY STRATEGIES FOR MASTERING THE MIND-BODY CONNECTION

Your attitude and outlook can have major effects on your health. The following tips, courtesy of Mental Health America (formerly the National Mental Health Association), may help you feel better in body, mind, and spirit.

1. Cultivate Your Positive Emotions.

WHY: According to research . . .

- Positive thinking can build emotional resilience and reduce stress.

- The simple act of laughing may deliver short-term physiological benefits like reduced anxiety and promote muscle relaxation.

- Optimistic people had an almost 20 percent lower risk of dying over a thirty-year period than people who were pessimistic.

- People who paused once a week to consider the things they were grateful for were happier and had less physical problems than others.

- When subjects wrote a "gratitude letter" thanking a person who'd been especially kind to them or had an important positive impact on their lives, and they delivered the letter in person, the letter writers enjoyed strong positive effects even a month later.

HOW:

- Pay attention to the risks and negatives of life, but focus on the positives as much as possible.

- Boost your optimism by writing down your vision of a beautiful future for you and your family, your goals, and dreams. They may not all come true but it's the pursuit and journey that builds optimism.

- Flip lousy situations into positives—focus on what you've learned and how the experience makes you smarter and stronger.

- Keep a gratitude journal. At least once a week, write down the things that make you smile—people you love, great news, big achievements, sweet little moments.

- Write thank-you letters to people who've had a positive impact on your life—and if you can, deliver them in person.

- Savor the good things in life. Grab all the roses you can find and inhale deeply!

- Don't over-obsess on the negatives. Change unhealthy self-talk. You may have been running negative messages in your head for a long time, but research shows that you can learn to shift your thoughts and that, over time, you can literally change your brain.

- Try to laugh at some of the hassles in your life, if possible. Finding what's a little absurd or amusing in a tough situation just might make it less painful.

- Learn some tips from cognitive-behavioral therapy, a highly effective technique used by psychiatrists that looks at how changing your thoughts can change your life. For example:

  - Is your negative thought really true?

  - Imagine what you'd tell a friend if she was worrying like you are now.

  - Beware of thinking things are all or nothing. One bad situation doesn't guarantee others.

- Take a nature break. Drink in the oxygen and sunlight of a power walk in the park.

- Practice mindfulness, or the experience of fully relishing all the little things as well as the big ones. Savor each bite of a meal, each funny thing your child does, each embrace you share with a loved one.

2. Strengthen Your Social Bonds

WHY? According to research . . .

- Good relationships can contribute to better health, increase happiness, and extend your life.

- People who regularly help others are calmer, less depressed, and healthier. They may even live longer.

- Students who performed five acts of altruism a day boosted their own feelings of happiness.

- Giving emotional support to other people can decrease the harmful health effects of stress.

- Brain imaging research revealed that people who gave money to charity got a boost in a feel-good part of the brain.

- Helping others can help you feel fortunate, needed, effective, and connected to others, and can add meaning and purpose to your life.

HOW:

- Plan a weekly date with your spouse.

- Reach out to old friends and colleagues. Catch up and cheer them on.

- Pump up your "pit crew"—the people you're closest to and feel the most comfortable and happy around.

- Create new networks. Get out there and make new friends and connections by joining clubs, groups, teams, and volunteer organizations.

- Volunteer at a food pantry, homeless shelter, school, hospital, clinic, tutoring/mentoring program, or center for children, immigrants, or veterans.

3. Nurture Your Spiritual Side

WHY? According to research . . .

- Spirituality may offer benefits like improving mood and reducing anxiety and depression.

- In one study, people with strong religious beliefs recovered faster from heart surgery than people with weaker faith.

- People who meditate have increased activity in a "feel good" area of the brain.

- Spirituality may help reduce the stress that can trigger or exacerbate illness, and can also provide a sense of purpose and meaning to your life.

HOW:

- For many people, spirituality means religious rituals, texts, and services. For others, it's about things they consider meaningful and holy. You might find spirituality in God, in yourself, in other people, in nature, or in love and compassion.

- If you're so inclined, join a religious institution. In general, people who attend a house of worship regularly may be happier and healthier, some research suggests, likely because of the social connection involved. This may also be because religious groups support healthy lifestyle choices, like reduced smoking and drinking.

- Pray or focus on your notion of God or whatever it is that you find strength in. You can pray from your own heart when you need some solace, and uttering a prayer of gratitude may improve your mood.

- Talk with others who share similar spiritual beliefs and learn from each other.

- Volunteer with a religious or spiritual group or charity.

- If more traditional prayers and practices are not for you (and even if they are), you might try meditation, which may deliver real health benefits.

- When appropriate, try to forgive—for your own sake. Research shows that forgiving reduces tension, depression and anxiety.

Courtesy of and adapted from Mental Health America http://liveyourlifewell.org

I once took care of an amazing woman who came to the ER on what turned out to be her last night on earth. She was suffering from terminal cancer and had developed a fever. She kept smiling whenever I entered her room, and all the while I could tell she knew her hours were numbered.

When I asked her how she could be so optimistic during such a tough time for her, she pointed to her family in the room and said, "I've lived a wonderful life and I have nothing to be sad about."

As I left her room for the last time she was still smiling. I will never forget her face. Any time I have a negative attitude, I always think back to her on that night. If she could smile in the face of such adversity—certain death—then how can I justify having a bad attitude when dealing with minor, everyday matters?

The moral of the story: Don't sweat the small stuff, and be grateful for every moment we have on Earth. It's an attitude that's good for our health—and for our souls.

DR. STORK'S ANTIAGING TIPS: 3 THINGS YOU CAN DO TODAY TO INCREASE YOUR LIFE SPAN AND YOUR QUALITY OF LIFE

Don't waste your money on expensive anti-aging pills or tonics. It's the simple things that are going to give you the biggest bang for your buck for your optimal wellness.

Aging well isn't just about the length of your life; it should primarily be about enjoying a healthy, disease-free, happy existence. After all, who wants to live to one hundred unless they're feeling great?

To live long, stay out of the hospital, and live a physically and mentally happy life, follow these simple, proven guidelines. If they sound familiar, they should—it ought to come as no surprise that the behaviors that will make you feel great are also the ones that will optimize your health. It's all connected.

1. Eat Healthy over the Long Term.

Eat to Savor Life. What you eat, and how much you eat, has a tremendous impact on how long and how well you will live.

2. Get Regular Physical Activity.

I've said it before and I'll say it again: few behaviors have as big an impact on your life span as physical activity. If you exercise, you will live longer.

3. Learn to Relax and Reduce Stress.

You can't always control what people do to you, but you can control how you react to it.

For example, a bad boss can wreak havoc on your health and infuse your life with a tremendous amount of stress. I recently read a study that suggested that the longer you have a bad boss, the higher your risk of heart attack. When we're in a stressful work situation, we experience physiological changes: our heart rates go up, and stress hormones cause us to have increased blood pressure, which makes our hearts work harder over time. That's why we have an increased risk of heart attack. And unfortunately, when people get stressed out, they can stop making healthy food choices, lose sleep, and things snowball in a very unhealthy direction.

Or consider what happens when you undergo a fight-or-flight response the night before a big test, or before a big presentation, or during a sudden major stressor like losing control of your car. Your mind feels fear and your body (in the form of your adrenal glands) releases epinephrine (aka adrenaline). Your heart rate and blood pressure go up, and you can start to sweat. You feel extremely nervous and anxious, but also hyperfocused. We need this natural fight-or-flight physiological response, because otherwise we'd never be motivated to accomplish much of anything. But too much stress—chronic stress—really is bad for us.

While short-term, acute stress allows us to focus on studying for that exam, chronic worry and stress causes our bodies to release too much of a hormone called cortisol (aka the stress hormone) and chronically elevated levels of cortisol are not good for us. Over time high levels can contribute to premature death, as our visceral fat levels (the fat around our internal organs in our abdomen) increase and our risk for diabetes, heart disease, and many other chronic diseases may also increase. How's that for a mind-body connection?

Here are my top three strategies for fighting stress, adapted from MHA:

1. Get up and get moving. Go for a jog, lift some weights, smack a tennis ball, do some yoga, or chase your kids or your dog around the yard. Exercise is a proven stress buster.

2. Switch off the electronic devices. Stop emailing and texting, and shut off the TV, the PDA, and the internet for a good chunk of your day. You'll feel it's much easier to mellow out when you're disconnected from all those sources of stress and eyestrain.

3. Tap into some instant karma. Try one of these three easy types of meditation, as described by the experts at Mental Health America:

- Deep Breathing

  - Sit or lie down comfortably.

  - Rest your hands on your stomach.

  - Slowly count to four while inhaling through your nose.

  - Feel your stomach rise.

  - Hold your breath for a second.

  - Slowly count to four while you exhale, preferably through pursed lips to control the breath.

  - Feel your stomach fall slowly. Repeat a few times.

- Mindfulness Meditation

  - Focus on your breath.

  - Notice anything that passes through your awareness without judgment.

  - If your mind starts to tackle your to-do list, return to focusing on your breath.

- Visualization

  - Close your eyes, relax, and imagine a peaceful place, like a forest. Engage all your senses: hear the crunching leaves, smell the damp soil, feel the breeze.

■ Repeat a mantra. Sit quietly and pick any meaningful or soothing word, phrase, or sound. You can repeat the mantra aloud or silently. Experts say the repetition creates a physical relaxation response.

Courtesy of and adapted from Mental Health America

Quick and Easy Takeaways for Mastering the Mind-Body Connection

- Your mind may be the single most important factor in your physical health. Your decisions, positive thinking, and commitment can transform your physical destiny and add decades of healthy living to your life.

- Mind-body therapies have benefits for our mental and physical health, and most are safe and easy to learn.

- Practices such as yoga, meditation, and Tai Chi are promising avenues to enhance our well-being, reduce stress, and aid in relaxation.

Epilogue

Congratulations, you have just completed a fantastic journey that will place you on the fast track to lasting good health.

You learned seven steps that, when put into action, will give you and your family a healthier, safer, and happier new life:

The 7-Step Prescription for Optimal Wellness

1. Be Your Own Health Guru.

2. Eat to Savor Life.

3. Give Your Body a Daily Physical Vacation.

4. Nail Your Health Stats.

5. Master the Medical Process.

6. Open Your Mind to Alternatives.

7. Make the Mind-Body Connection.

Go out and celebrate by taking someone you love out for a healthy, delicious meal, followed by a brisk, thirty-minute power walk!

The fact that you've made it through the book, that you've absorbed all of this important information and kept an open mind to the expert opinions and theories I've presented, tells me a lot about you.

It tells me you're ready to become your own health guru and make health your hobby.

It tells me you're ready to commit to optimal wellness, to putting these seven steps into action and to sticking with them for the long haul.

It tells me that from this moment on, you're ready to wake up every morning with a vision of a healthy life for you and your family, to take that destiny into your own hands and make it happen.

No book can hope to cover the entire universe of health information out there, but the seven steps I've outlined in these pages are the simplest, most powerful megastrategies you can use to achieve the best health possible.

If you fall into unhealthy habits once in a while, don't get discouraged. It happens to all of us. Some people can get really excited about making positive lifestyle changes, but they find the follow-through can be tough. The key is to stay positive and motivated and realize that a few unhealthy days here and there are not a reason to fall off the wagon because you can still be healthy in the long run.

Life is a complex existence, we have good days and bad days, joyful days and stressful days. You often can't control your life circumstances, but you can always control how you treat your body. And it all starts with your mental commitment to treating your body as well as you can.

I have one final request. I'd like you to get some Post-its and go back to the Quick and Easy Takeaway pages at the end of each of the seven chapters in this book and tag them, so whenever you get discouraged or you feel yourself falling off the wagon, you can remind yourself of the shortcuts for getting back on track.

One thing I've learned in my own life is that feeling healthy is a self-reinforcing cycle of positivity. When you change your mindset to treat your body right, and you stick to it, you'll slowly but surely over time feel better and better. When you start taking care of yourself, you see the world in a new and different way. You're more positive. Feeling better physically will make you feel better mentally and will give you the energy to stay on the right path. It's a fantastic payoff. Maybe it will take a week, two weeks, or a few months, but you will get there if you stick to it.

Whenever you need a pep talk, just tune in to *The Doctors* and I promise to always do my best to motivate you and practice what I preach. I, like you, am hardly perfect, and this is a lifelong, healthy journey that we're on together. I don't want to see you in my ER— I would much rather see you in our audience!

Until then, I wish you and your family the most love and energy possible, the best health, and the happiest life.

And remember, every morning when you wake up, you have the power to positively affect your life and health by making very simple but smart choices.

Acknowledgments

I thank these people for their valuable contributions to making this book a reality: William Doyle for his passion and for helping me translate my thoughts about optimal health into a living, breathing manuscript. My manager and friend, Lisa Furnish. Mel Berger and Kathy Armistead of William Morris Endeavor. Emily Westlake at Gallery Books and her colleagues Jennifer Weidman and Nancy Inglis. My colleagues at Vanderbilt University Medical Center and *The Doctors*, especially Jay McGraw, Andrew Scher, Carla Pennington, Dr. Phil McGraw, Dr. Jim Sears, Dr. Lisa Masterson, and Dr. Andrew Ordon. David Grotto, RD, and Karen Collins, RD, for reviewing and commenting on the healthy eating sections of the book.

Index

Note: Italic page numbers refer to illustrations.

About the Author

DR. TRAVIS STORK is a faculty physician in the Emergency Department at Vanderbilt Medical Center in Nashville, Tennessee, and host of the Emmy-nominated daily TV series *The Doctors*.

He graduated magna cum laude from Duke University and earned his MD with honors from the University of Virginia. He completed his residency as an emergency medicine doctor at Vanderbilt University.

WILLIAM DOYLE is an award-winning *New York Times* bestselling writer based in New York. Once clinically obese, he has maintained an over-thirty-pound weight loss for seven years through healthy eating and regular exercise.